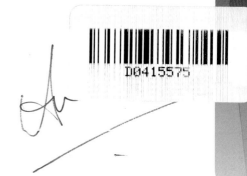

CLINICAL GOVERNANCE

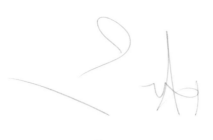

Commissioning Editor: Timothy Horne
Project Development Manager: Siân Jarman
Project Manager: Nancy Arnott
Designer: Erik Bigland
Illustrator: MTG

CLINICAL GOVERNANCE

John Wright
Associate Medical Director
Bradford Royal Infirmary, Bradford

Peter Hill
Postgraduate Dean and Director for
Postgraduate Institute of Medicine and Dentistry
University of Newcastle upon Tyne
Newcastle upon Tyne

Foreword by
Sir Liam Donaldson
Chief Medical Officer

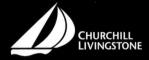

CHURCHILL
LIVINGSTONE

EDINBURGH LONDON NEW YORK PHILADELPHIA ST LOUIS SYDNEY
TORONTO 2003

PREFACE

Times are changing in medicine. In the past the assumption has been that medical care is effective, safe, the doctor knows everything and the patients do as we say. We have woken up to the fact that a lot of medicine is not effective, frequently unsafe and that our learning as doctors does not stop at graduation, but continues all our professional lives. Patients have become much more informed and empowered and have become increasingly consumerist in their approach to health care.

In the past, the quality of care that we provide for patients has been left to us as individuals. As a result, standards of practice have been variable and attempts to improve the quality of health care have often been haphazard, undervalued and covert.

Clinical governance has changed our approach to ensuring that patients receive the best possible care. It recognizes the importance of teams, organizations and systems in health care rather than individuals working in isolation. It provides a framework for tying together the different strands of quality – audit and feedback, clinical effectiveness, error reduction and risk management, evidence-based practice, patient involvement and lifelong learning. It places a statutory responsibility on senior managers to promote a culture where quality rather than money is the priority in the health service.

In the past, quality of care and clinical governance would have remained in the realm of the few, and at the margins for the majority. Now it is at the heart of all our work as doctors. This book describes what clinical governance is and how it works in practice. It dismantles the building blocks and demonstrates how to construct quality improvement from scratch. It provides an action guide to clinical governance with case histories, practical examples and clear explanations to help bring this important subject to life for the reader. We hope it will equip and inspire medical students, and junior and senior doctors to take the first step onto the quality escalator.

We owe a debt of gratitude to many people who have helped with this book. We would like to thank everybody who has contributed support and ideas, in particular Margaret Haigh, Mike Smith, Derek Tuffnell, Tony Roberts, Chris Cates, colleagues at the Postgraduate Institute and all the staff at Bradford Hospitals Trust. We owe much more to our families for their encouragement and nurturing.

Bradford   J. W
Newcastle   P. H
2003

FOREWORD

Two senior doctors meet in the corridor of their hospital on Monday morning. Both are busy but cannot resist stopping for a short conversation. One explains that she has come up with an idea for significantly improving the process of care for patients with diabetes mellitus. The other doctor becomes very excited as he immediately sees the potential for improved outcomes of care and a more convenient way for patients to receive support and advice.

They agree to take the idea to the Friday morning multidisciplinary clinical governance meeting where opportunities for quality improvements are discussed, analysed and planned. The first consultant agrees to talk to the nurse consultant in diabetology, the patient representative in that area of service and the lead local general practitioner in diabetes management and ask them whether they would be able to join Friday's discussion.

Traditionally corridor conversations between clinical colleagues have often been about particular patient care problems – perhaps agreeing to talk further about a difficult diagnosis or treatment options. Too often in the last ten years as volume and complexity of work has grown, more conversations have been about the negatives of professional life.

Health services are striving to create the kinds of organization where a passion for quality is instilled throughout the organization. Where all staff have a curiosity, a drive, an enthusiasm for innovation and improvement. Where solving individual clinical problems is still vital but where seeing opportunities for better care for hundreds of patients captures the imagination of all staff.

That is the dream. Making it a reality means infusing all NHS organizations, all clinical teams, all individual practitioners with the principles of clinical governance. This means creating health care organizations where the culture, systems and infrastructure are fully patient centred and build in a dynamic for quality assurance and quality improvement as part of their every day functioning.

John Wright and Peter Hill have written a highly authoritative, comprehensive and accessible book on clinical governance. It will be of great value to those with responsibility for implementing clinical governance within their own health care organizations as well as students and others who want to find out what clinical governance is all about and what it means in practice.

This book is an important and timely work which deserves to be widely read.

Sir Liam Donaldson
Chief Medical Officer
Department of Health

CONTENTS

Introduction

Clinical governance is 'a framework through which NHS organizations are accountable for continuously improving the quality of their services and safeguarding high standards of care by creating an environment in which excellence in clinical care will flourish'.[1] A statutory duty for quality was placed on all NHS (National Health Service) organizations in the Health Act 1999.

This chapter covers:

- The historical perspective
- The concept of clinical governance
- Quality assurance in health care
- Total quality management and other models
- The global perspective
- Developing clinical governance
- The National Institute for Clinical Excellence
- The Commission for Health Audit and Inspection
- National standards
- Clinical governance for doctors, including revalidation and appraisal
- The characteristics of an ideal health service.

THE HISTORICAL PERSPECTIVE

The term governance was derived from the commercial world following a number of high profile institutional failures with significant losses of investor funds. Corporate governance is the system by which companies are directed and controlled. Boards of directors are responsible for the governance of their companies. The shareholders' role is to appoint the directors and the auditors, and to satisfy themselves that appropriate arrangements for governance are in place. It is the responsibility of the board to set the strategic aims for the company and provide the leadership to put them into effect. The board also has to supervise the management of the business and report to the shareholders on their stewardship. The actions of the board are subject to laws and regulations, and to the shareholders, such as at an annual general meeting.

So it is with hospital and health care trusts.

In relation to hospitals the term is much older, going back to 1660,[2] and it has been argued that we can go back to Hippocrates in 400 BC to find that the medical profession has operated some form of clinical governance.

THE CONCEPT

Clinical governance is therefore largely a new name for established concepts. It can be viewed as a whole system cultural change which provides the means of developing organizational capability to deliver sustainable, accountable, patient-focused, quality-assured health care.

Recent events

More recently, in the 1990s and early part of the new millennium, there have been some widely reported spectacular failures of medical care in England. These have included catastrophic failings in screening services for breast and cervical cancer, the public inquiry into the excessive number of deaths of babies treated surgically for heart problems at the Bristol Royal Infirmary, individual doctors who have served considerable numbers of patients badly leading to damage and harm, and the infamous Dr Shipman, a general practitioner who murdered large numbers of his patients over many years.

In what is likely to become a seminal moment, the report of the Bristol inquiry into children's heart surgery covering a period of 10 years from mid-1980 to the middle of 1990 identified over 30 children under the age of 1 year who died unnecessarily, and many more were injured.[3] The report acknowledged that the whole NHS had failed to change with the times. The NHS was described as having no system for monitoring quality, no reliable data, and no agreement about what constituted quality. Nearly 200 recommendations were made (Box 1.1).[3]

Box 1.1   Requirements of the NHS specified by the Bristol report

There needs to be:

- Patients put first
- Good leadership
- A better system of accountability
- Better management
- Better communication
- Public involvement at all levels.

(Adapted from: Public Inquiry into Children's Heart Surgery at the Bristol Royal Infirmary 1984–1995. *Learning from Bristol*. London: Stationery Office, 2001 (Cmnd 5207).)

QUALITY ASSURANCE IN HEALTH CARE

There is a substantial literature, mostly from North America, on the difficult issue of defining quality in health care. Donabedian is rightly credited with the pioneering classification of structure, process, and the outcome of care[4] (Box 1.2). However, not all of this work is covered with glory.

Systematic audit, for example, was pioneered in America by a surgeon, Ernest Codman, in the early part of the last century. Codman raised the

Introduction

Box 1.2   Donabedian's model of health care quality

The model is based on:

Structure: The physical features of health care, e.g. equipment, resources
Process: What happens to patients, e.g. clinical examinations, prescriptions
Outcomes: The change in health status that can be attributed to the preceding health care

---

(Adapted from: Donabedian A. Evaluating the quality of medical care. *Milbank Memorial Fund Quarterly* 1966; **4**: 166–206.)

---

possibility of linking outcome after surgery to the process of care. Codman believed that hospital care could be standardized and related to the process of care in hospital, and he suggested an independent agency to act as a regulating body. From this idea was born the American College of Surgeons, and this was formed in 1912. Surgeons in practice could not devote enough time to this work, so a capable administrator who was not medically qualified, John G. Bowman, was appointed to oversee the formidable task of introducing audit. There were some 2700 hospitals to be surveyed. Bowman planned to use objective criteria to analyse the salient stages in the diagnosis, clinical management and outcomes of treatments. However, when this was put to the test only 89 out of 692 hospitals with 100 beds or more could meet any reasonable standard. There is a graphic description of how the facts elicited by the first survey were so shocking that a committee ordered the original survey data to be destroyed immediately. The draft report and the database were burned by the Regents of the American College of Surgeons in the furnace of the Waldorf Astoria Hotel in New York in October 1919.[5]

Other models of quality in health care

Maxwell has offered a model based on six dimensions of health care quality (Box 1.3):[6]

- Accessibility: is a service accessible to the people it is designed to serve? This means in terms of both physical accessibility, and the time it takes to get there.
- Relevance to need: are the services or procedures what the population and individuals need?

Box 1.3   Dimensions of health care quality

Access to services
Relevance to need for the whole community
Effectiveness for individual patients
Equity (fairness)
Social acceptability
Efficiency and economy

(Adapted from: Maxwell RJ. Quality assessment in health. *BMJ* 1984; **288**: 1470–1472.)

- Effectiveness: does the service achieve its intended or desired benefits or outcomes for individuals or groups of patients?
- Equity: is the service provided fairly between different patients and client groups?
- Social acceptability: are the conditions in which the service is provided, the arrangements for privacy, the level of communication with patients, family and carers, etc. satisfactory?
- Efficiency: are resources used without waste?

Some people add a further dimension, that of safety. This aspect would question whether the service and health professionals and staff providing it take all steps to minimize adverse effects of treatment. Other dimensions could be added. It has been argued that respect, choice, and the availability of information should be included in any definition.

The priorities given to different principles in any model will depend on the different imperatives of the different stakeholders. These would include the recipients of the service or treatment, those professionals who refer patients to the service, the health professionals and staff involved in providing the service, managers, and the payers (taxpayers, through the Government with funding routed via health authorities and health care trusts).

TOTAL QUALITY MANAGEMENT

Total quality management (TQM, also referred to as continuous quality improvement or CQI) refers to a management process directed at establishing organized continuous improvement activities, involving everyone in an organization in a totally integrated effort towards improving performance at every level. TQM is really a management philosophy and business strategy with roots in the work of US and Japanese strategists, such as Demming. The four general ideas underpinning TQM are:

- Organizational success relies on every department meeting the needs of those it serves (customers) and many of these customers will be internal to the organization;
- Quality is an effect caused by the processes of production in which the causal systems are complex but understandable;
- Most human beings engaged in work are intrinsically motivated to try hard and do well, and;
- Simple statistical methods linked with careful collection and analysis of data on work processes can yield powerful insights into the causes of problems within those work processes.

The focus of TQM is on processes of work, rather than the workers themselves. The aim is that changes are introduced steadily and forever to improve quality. The implementation of TQM involves:

- A focus on work processes – not just providing clear direction about the expected outcomes; management must train and coach employees to assess, analyse and improve work processes.

- Explicit identification and measurement of customer requirements (internal and external).
- Analysis of variations – uncontrolled variations in processes or outcomes are the primary cause of quality problems, and must be analysed and controlled by those who do the work.
- Teams who cross the various functions are needed to identify and solve quality problems.
- Management by fact – the use of systematically collected data at every point in a problem-solving cycle involving high priority problems, analysing their causes, and selecting and testing solutions or changes.
- Learning and continuous improvement – treating quality as a never-ending quest.
- Using process management tools to enhance team effectiveness, e.g. flow charts, brainstorming, cause and effect diagrams and benchmarking.

Business process re-engineering

Business process re-engineering (BPR) is a technique employed to change the organization and came to prominence in the early 1990s. The main concepts that underpin the BPR approach include:

- Organizations should be organized around key processes rather than specialist functions.
- Narrow specialists should be replaced by multi-skilled workers, often working in self-managed teams.
- In contrast with incremental techniques like TQM, BPR involves a total change from current practices and radical rethinking.
- The direction for the required radical rethinking comes unequivocally from top management.

An example of improving quality through process redesign is shown in Box 1.4.

Box 1.4   Improving quality through process redesign – an example

Staff in an endoscopy clinic of a large acute hospital were concerned about the quality of service provided and set about to improve the process of care. A small project multidisciplinary team (doctor, nurse, manager, secretary and GP) was established and three steps were followed.

Understanding the current process through a mapping exercise of referral pathways, attendance rates, clinic administration and a description of the patient pathway from staff and patient feedback and views.

Results. Delays were identified between receipt of the referral letter and sending out of appointments. There were long waits for appointments. 10% of sessions were cancelled, and 20% of patients failed to attend. 40% of patients were considered as inappropriate referrals. Staff complained of spending too much time chasing notes and results. Patients complained of lack of information and anxiety over the procedure.

Designing a new process. The project team then set about planning changes to improve quality. Information was gathered from other units in the country to find examples of best

---

practice and compare standards. The team then spent protected time brainstorming ideas and developing an ideal service.

Results. There was streamlining of administration with appointments sent out on the same day the referral was received. Targets were set for waiting times and clinic cancellations. Clinical assistants were trained to provide more sessions. Greater flexibility over appointments and the introduction of booked appointments. Better information for patients before and after endoscopy, with a contact number for queries. Referral guidelines developed in collaboration with primary care supported by educational sessions.

Implementation and review. There was a major reduction in administrative delays, waiting times and non-attendance rates. Appropriateness of referrals improved and patient satisfaction also increased.

Setting targets for each of the changes has allowed progress to be regularly monitored and fed back to staff. The team approach fostered a more positive working environment and shared goals that have provided a sustainable approach to continuous quality improvement.

THE GLOBAL PERSPECTIVE

The concern with quality is global. In 1985 the World Health Organization (WHO) set a target that, 'By 1990, all Member States should have built effective mechanisms for ensuring the quality of patient care within their health care systems'.[7] The principles have been defined by WHO and must include at least four dimensions (Box 1.5).[8] These four dimensions are professional performance, resource use, risk management and patient satisfaction with services provided. Any quality assurance programme, in the view of WHO, must ensure that each patient receives such a mix of diagnostic and therapeutic health services as is most likely to produce the optimal achievable health care outcome for that patient, consistent with the state of the art of medical science, and with biological factors (such as the patient's age, illness, concomitant secondary diagnoses, compliance with treatment); with the minimal expenditure of resources necessary to accomplish this result; at the lowest achievable risk of additional injury or disability as a consequence of the treatment; and with maximal patient satisfaction with the process of care, his or her interaction with the health care system, and the results obtained.

Box 1.5   Dimensions of quality

Professional performance: technical quality

Resource use: economic efficiency

Risk management: the identification and avoidance of injury, harm or illness associated with the service provided

Patient satisfaction

(Adapted from: WHO Working Group. The principles of quality assurance. *Quality Assurance in Health Care* 1989; **1**: 79–95.)

Why clinical governance is needed

Clinical governance is required because of the increasing public and governmental intolerance of what are perceived to be repeated inadequacies and consistently poor standards of care in the National Health Service. There needs to be a mechanism for public accountability for the delivery of health services, not least because of the large sums of public money involved.

This leads to a managerial dimension, since there is a responsibility, in being publicly accountable, to identify and solve problems. This means that clinical governance approaches must be embedded in each clinical department or general practice as part of their general responsibilities.

Clinical governance is also needed because of well documented widespread evidence of variations in care, and to prevent inappropriate care (Figure 1.1).[9,10] There is also a large body of evidence to indicate that iatrogenic disease is substantial. It is important to remember that any resource used in one way is not available for use in some other way. Thus, if resources are used ineffectively or inefficiently, then other patients will be denied the opportunity to benefit. There are thus social and economic motives for clinical governance, to ensure that potential benefits to patients can be maximized, and that unnecessary risks can be avoided.

Other drivers for quality

But there are other drivers for better quality. Professional motives are of key importance. Most health professionals are altruistic and keen to do their best for patients. One of the elements of being a professional is having a self-questioning attitude, with a desire to be self-correcting and self-regulating.

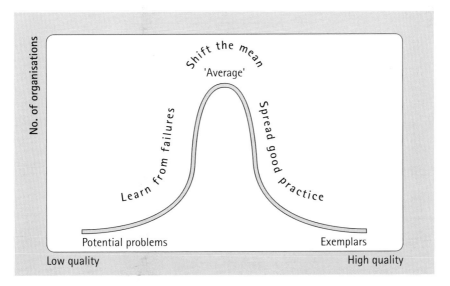

Fig. 1.1 Variation in the quality of health organizations. (Adapted from: Scally G, Donaldson LJ. Clinical governance and the drive for quality improvement in the new NHS in England. *BMJ* 1998; **317**: 61–65.)

Indeed, intellectual curiosity may be aroused in relation to analysing and explaining differences in patterns of practice and the results of care or service provision. Much professional satisfaction derives from being involved in identifying where improvements can be made and taking steps to effect these. This is part of identifying one's own educational needs.

The concept of clinical governance is one whose simplicity belies the underlying complexity. It would be difficult to conceive of anyone among the public, professionals, or paymasters in government who would not subscribe wholeheartedly to notions of a high quality national health service.

One of the key characteristics of clinical governance that is likely to ensure its endurance is its all pervading nature. Clinical governance embraces not only patients and health professionals, but also managerial colleagues and policy makers. It is a top to bottom cultural phenomenon.

DEVELOPING CLINICAL GOVERNANCE

The promotion of the statutory duty for quality through clinical governance as the backbone of the quest for excellence throughout the health service is supported by a number of different policy strands operating at different levels (see Figure 1.2).[1] The key elements of the NHS quality strategy have been defined (see Box 1.6). There are also a number of national structures and processes, as well as approaches that focus on the performance of individual health professionals.

Structures in place include the National Institute for Clinical Excellence, the Commission for Health Audit and Inspection and the National Clinical Assessment Authority.

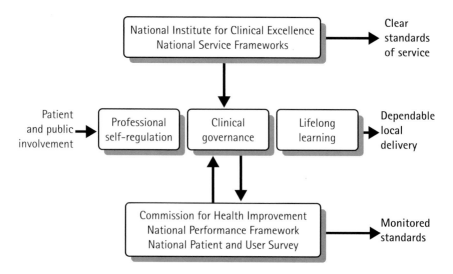

Fig. 1.2 Setting, delivering and monitoring standards. (Adapted from: Department of Health. A First Class Service: quality in the new NHS. Health Service Circular: HSC(98)113. London: Department of Health, 1998.)

Introduction

Box 1.6   Key elements of the quality strategy

- Standards:
  - National Institute for Clinical Excellence
  - National Service Frameworks
- Local duty of quality:
  - Clinical governance
  - Controls assurance
- Assuring quality of individual practice:
  - NHS performance procedures
  - Annual appraisal
  - Revalidation
- Scrutiny:
  - Commission for Health Audit and Inspection
  - Education inspection visits
- Learning mechanisms:
  - Adverse incident reporting
  - Learning networks
  - Continuing professional development
- Patient empowerment:
  - Better information
  - New patient advocacy service
  - Rights of redress
  - Patients' views sought
  - Patients involved throughout the NHS
- Underpinning strategies:
  - Information and information technology
  - Research and development
  - Education and training

(Adapted from: Halligan A, Donaldson L. Implementing clinical governance: turning vision into reality. *BMJ* 2001; **322**: 1413–1417.)

THE NATIONAL INSTITUTE FOR CLINICAL EXCELLENCE (NICE)

NICE (*www.nice.org.uk*) is a Special Health Authority that was set up in 1999 to provide clinicians with evidence of best practice and advice on which treatments work best and are most cost-effective for patients. The reasons for its establishment stem from concerns over cost pressures for new and expensive drugs and technologies; variation in practices leading to 'postcode rationing' and the perceived need for authoritative guidance to inform a high quality NHS. It has three main roles.

Health technology appraisal

National guidance is given on the clinical effectiveness and cost-effectiveness of new and existing health technologies. These include drugs, investigations and operations. The aim is to reduce so-called 'postcode' prescribing where patients receive new drugs or treatments in one health district, but can be refused them in a neighbouring district.

Examples of NICE appraisals include:

- Guidance on the clinical and cost-effectiveness of inhaler devices in asthma.
- Guidance on the use of new drugs such as interferon beta for multiple sclerosis and proton pump inhibitors.
- Guidance on the use of laparoscopic surgery for inguinal hernia.
- Guidance on the removal of wisdom teeth.

Clinical guideline development

Many guidelines that are developed in hospitals or health districts are of variable quality. Guidelines on the same topic often give contradictory or divergent advice. NICE is producing national guidelines on specific clinical topics such as breast cancer, schizophrenia, dyspepsia, diabetes and multiple sclerosis.

Promotion of clinical audit and confidential inquiries

Guidance from NICE can be complemented with advice about standards and methods for clinical audit. This is to allow clinicians to measure how well they are performing in chosen areas such as acute low back pain, stroke and myocardial infarction. The four National Confidential Enquiries are also incorporated under the NICE umbrella.

NICE guidance is published on a variety of different topics at regular intervals. Each hospital or health care organization should ensure that it has an effective system for disseminating this guidance and subsequently auditing practice to demonstrate adherence with recommendations.

NICE provides technology appraisals and clinical guidelines for health professionals in England and Wales. In Scotland, the Scottish Intercollegiate Guidelines Network (SIGN) develops and disseminates national clinical guidelines. SIGN was formed in 1993 with a multidisciplinary membership and has a strong track record in developing evidence-based guidelines.

The Health Technology Board for Scotland (*www.htbs.org.uk*) undertakes a similar role to NICE in providing guidance on the clinical and cost-effectiveness of new drugs and technologies.

SUPPORT FOR CLINICAL GOVERNANCE

The NHS Clinical Governance Support Team (*www.ncgst.nhs.uk*) was established in 1999 to support the development and implementation of clinical governance. It aims to promote the goals of clinical governance across the NHS; to act as a focus of expertise, advice and information; and to offer a training and development programme for clinical teams and NHS organizations.

Development programmes are run over a series of learning days for multidisciplinary teams. Delegates return to their organizations between learning days and try to design and implement quality improvement programmes in their clinical area. Programmes use a RAID[11] (review, agree, implement, demonstrate) model to promote good project management.

The Clinical Governance Support Team reinforces this work with front-line clinicians by working with NHS hospitals and organizations. Visits are undertaken to help Trust boards promote and support an open culture for dissemination and uptake of clinical governance initiatives.

THE COMMISSION FOR HEALTH AUDIT AND INSPECTION (CHAI)

The Commission for Health Audit and Inspection (*www.chai.nhs.uk*) is an independent body that was set up in 1999 following recommendations in the *First-Class Service* white paper. Its main role is to undertake clinical governance reviews every 4–5 years in all primary and secondary care organizations in the NHS.

CHAI also has a role in reviewing standards of care in organizations where there have been major service failures, undertaking studies of the impact and implementation of National Service Frameworks, and developing leadership and clinical governance capacity in the health service. In the past, when there have been failures in whole clinical services or NHS organizations (such as with Bristol's paediatric heart surgery) the subsequent enquiries have often been disparate and inconsistent. CHAI has now taken on this role of external investigation in the place of other bodies such as the Royal Colleges or NHS Trusts themselves. Examples of such enquiries undertaken by CHAI include investigation of abuse of elderly patients in North Lakeland Trust; high mortality from heart and lung transplantation at St George's Trust; removal of the wrong kidney at the Carmarthenshire Trust.

What is assessed

CHAI's model for assessment of Hospital and Primary Care Trusts is shown in Figure 1.3.[11] Clinical governance is broken down into seven 'technical' components:

- Consultation and patient involvement
- Clinical risk management
- Education, training and professional development
- Clinical audit
- Research and effectiveness
- Staffing and staff management
- Use of information about patients' experiences.

Each component is judged on a four-point scale (1 = poor, 4 = excellent). Organizational components for assessment by CHAI include managerial and clinical leadership, patient/public partnership, resources for quality improvement and staff focus.

A CHAI review takes place in three stages (see Box 1.7). The CHAI reviews are intended to be developmental rather than judgmental – the review is

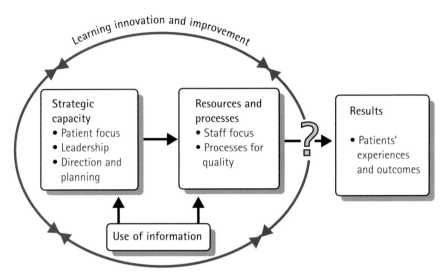

Fig. 1.3 The CHAI model for clinical governance. (Adapted from: Bevan G, Bawden D. Clinical data and information, and clinical governance. *Clinical Governance Bulletin* 2001; **2**: 2–3.)

Box 1.7 The three stages of a CHAI review

Pre-visit preparation | This involves extensive data collection about all clinical governance activity in the Trust. Information requested will vary from Trust Board minutes and strategic plans to lists of complaints for previous years. A self-assessment report is submitted outlining clinical strengths and weaknesses in the Trust. This identifies up to five departments with best and worst clinical governance practice.

Hospital activity is extensively analysed for information on admissions, length of stay, operations, mortality and maternity outcomes.

Other health organizations (PCTs, Health Authority, Community Health Council, patient groups) are also invited to participate. Stakeholder meetings are held to obtain the views of local people.

Based on the data collection and recommendations from the Trust, three clinical departments are selected for site review. This usually comprises a mixture of identified good practice and potential weak areas with outlying performance.

Hospital or site visit | A multidisciplinary team undertakes a site visit. This comprises a doctor, a nurse, a lay member, a manager, one other health professional and one review manager. The first 3 days are spent with the three chosen teams, fact-finding, interviewing and observing. The final 2 days are spent interviewing senior staff and board members.

Reporting | Debriefing by review team. Report writing. Subsequent objective setting and action plan in the light of review recommendations. A workshop is organized to discuss the report and agree local objectives.

supposed to be a mirror held in front of the organization reflecting the best and the worst quality of care. So hospitals should not expect to receive a four star, or four stethoscope, grading to hang outside the main entrance. Rather areas are identified where improvements could be made or where there is substandard care. The action plan then details how improvements can be made. These are subsequently reviewed by the Strategic Health Authority and the Regional Directorate of Health and Social Care. So whether the quality of care in the organization is excellent or poor, the outcome from a CHAI visit will be to raise standards.

There are a number of potential negative elements of a CHAI visit:

- There are no clear standards by which they assess the different components of clinical governance and in most cases there is no obviously 'right' way of doing things.
- Although it is intended to be developmental the review can feel very much like an inspection and judgement.
- Rather than engendering partnership the review can lead to staff feeling threatened and resentful of the scrutiny and intrusion.
- The amount of data required by CHAI and the administration necessary to organize all the interviews during the visit can become a bureaucratic nightmare.
- The review can be time-consuming for clinical staff with opportunity costs for patient care.
- The quality of the review is very dependent on the quality of the review team and this will inevitably be variable, particularly as the NHS has not nurtured appropriate skills in its staff in the past.

What can be done in preparation?

Attempts to decorate and portray clinical governance development as something that it is not would defeat the purpose of real quality improvement, and would also be obvious to the reviewers. So resist any impulse to take up a creative writing course in clinical governance. At the same time, rather than being frozen in the oncoming CHAI headlights, there are steps that clinical departments should take to review their clinical governance arrangements in the run up to a visit:

- Promote awareness of the assessment and its components to staff. All staff should be clear about how they will be evaluated.
- Review their clinical governance arrangements against the assessment components (*www.chai.nhs.uk*) to identify strengths and weaknesses, describe where clinical governance has led to changes and improvements and review current departmental objectives.
- Review patient and public involvement in each department. This is a particularly important area for the CHAI review, not just in ensuring patient involvement, but also that patients' views shape current and future services.
- Collate all relevant clinical governance documents for the department from previous years for sending to CHAI during the pre-visit information gathering. A checklist can facilitate this.

NATIONAL CLINICAL ASSESSMENT AUTHORITY

Where individual doctors are believed to be demonstrating evidence of poor clinical performance, early referral to the National Clinical Assessment Authority (NCAA) is expected, in order to reduce any risks to patients. It is the role of the NCAA to make a thorough and objective assessment, and provide advice to the NHS employer.

THE CLINICAL STANDARDS BOARD FOR SCOTLAND

In Scotland, the Clinical Standards Board for Scotland (*www.clinicalstandards.org*) has responsibility for external scrutiny and review of clinical quality in the health service. Its aims are:

- to promote public confidence that the services provided by the NHS are safe and that they meet nationally agreed standards and
- to demonstrate that, within the resources available, the NHS is delivering the highest possible standards of care.

The Board develops an annual programme of services to be reviewed, with opportunities for those within the NHS and the public to put forward suggestions. Initial priorities have been national priorities of cancer, coronary heart disease/stroke and mental health.

For each service the Board appoints a multidisciplinary project team including health care professionals and members of the public. These groups oversee the quality assurance and accreditation process: developing and consulting on the standards, managing external peer review, and reporting the conclusions to the Board.

NATIONAL STANDARDS

The key process for defining an explicit set of national standards to govern the delivery of health services at a local level are the National Service Frameworks (NSFs). NSFs set standards and targets as well as describing models of best practice. NSFs in place cover the investigation, diagnosis and management of cancer; coronary heart disease; mental health; and the care of older people. Others, including the care of children, are under development.

REVALIDATION AND APPRAISAL

The move towards more effective procedures also applies to the professional practice and performance of individual doctors. The General Medical Council (GMC) is undergoing major reforms to its structure and functions, to ensure enhanced accountability, more transparency, greater involvement of patients, and faster, more responsive procedures to protect patients from seriously

> **Box 1.8   Doing the right thing – two questions**
>
> • What would you do if, as a house officer, one of your colleagues turns up to an evening hand-over smelling of alcohol?
>
> Most junior doctors would know to take the colleague aside and quite rightly tell him or her to go home.
>
> • What would you do if, as a house officer, your consultant is called in during the evening smelling of alcohol?
>
> Most junior doctors, wrongly, would do nothing. However, silence and inaction are not acceptable responses in dealing with concerns over performance.

poor medical performance. Proposals are being developed for new 5-yearly checks and formal renewal of a doctor's licence to practice. This process is called revalidation.

Revalidation moves much further than processes largely established in other countries. These approaches are usually based on recertification or re-accreditation through passing examinations or other tests of competence. Revalidation moves the focus to an assessment of performance in the context of the job that the doctor does. Postgraduate deans are responsible for recommending revalidation of doctors in training.

The prime purpose of revalidation is to reassure the public that their doctors are competent and abide by high ethical standards (Box 1.8). Revalidation, as the culmination of an ongoing review of professional performance, is also meant to aid doctors in developing their skills. The stages involved include collecting evidence of competence and performance, regular reviews of the evidence, and having a group of medical and lay people make recommendations for revalidation, or referral to the GMC for a review of the doctor's registration.

Revalidation is linked to NHS appraisal, which has been in place for all health professionals since 1 April 2000.

Appraisal is an integral part of training and professional development for today's doctors and has become a standard requirement for GMC revalidation and a contractual agreement of employment. It is also an essential part of clinical governance, as it allows an opportunity to review an individual's work and performance, chart their continuing progress and identify development needs. It is intended to be formative, developmental, supportive, and linked to the requirement for continuing professional development. Therefore all doctors need a personal development plan.

Traditional appraisal has focused on reviewing achievements and developing an individual's performance in their work and is intended to be a positive experience. It should be a constructive dialogue for reflection and consideration as to how an individual can improve. Unfortunately this traditional role has been somewhat tortured and battered to become part of revalidation, and most doctors would now view the process as part of inevitable external assessment aimed at identifying the few doctors performing poorly rather than supporting the vast majority of doctors who are performing well.

Appraisal has a number of aims for both NHS employer and the individual to:

- Review clinical performance and obtain feedback
- Improve personal and professional effectiveness
- Discuss contributions to clinical governance and local priorities
- Identify learning needs and set future objectives
- Provide an opportunity for support and counselling.

GMC revalidation requirements set out a standardized format for appraisal. This involves every doctor maintaining an appraisal folder containing personal details, a current job description and documentation of evidence and information on clinical performance over the previous year. This should include recorded information on:

- Clinical workload
- Clinical governance activity
- Complaints, compliments and patient feedback
- Continuing professional development
- Relations with teams and colleagues
- Teaching and research activity.

Before the appraisal meeting, time should be invested in preparation. The doctor being appraised should reflect on the following questions:

- How good am I?
- How well do I perform?
- How up to date am I?
- How well do I work as part of a team?
- What resources and support do I need?
- How well am I meeting my service objectives?
- What are my development needs?

Appraisers need to be appropriately selected and adequately trained. Clinical directors and medical directors have crucial roles in appraisal of consultants, trainers have crucial roles in appraisal of trainees. Although the appraiser will vary, the skills needed in appraisal will not. A good appraiser needs to have the confidence of the appraisee, to be a good listener, to provide positive feedback support and to handle negative feedback constructively and sensitively.

THE IDEAL HEALTH SERVICE

The characteristics of an ideal health service have been defined (Box 1.9).[12] The challenge is to create an environment that fosters and rewards health care that is evidence-based, facilitated by a sophisticated information technology, where quality is rewarded, and where the workforce is prepared for rapid change in the interest of better service to patients. In our National Health Service, the patient's needs should drive the system, not the other way round. Clinical governance is central to this notion of a quality service, where quality

> **Box 1.9   The key characteristics of ideal health care**
>
> Safe: avoiding injuries to patients
>
> Effective: based on scientific knowledge (avoiding overuse and underuse)
>
> Patient-centred: respectful of and responsive to individuals' preferences, needs and values
>
> Timely: reducing wasteful delays
>
> Efficient: avoiding waits
>
> Equitable: the same quality of care provided to all, regardless of race, gender, geographic location, or ability to pay
>
> ---
>
> (After: Committee on Quality of Health Care in America. *Crossing the Quality Chasm: A New Health System for the 21st Century.* Washington, DC: National Academy Press, 2001. In: Kelly MA, Tucci JM. Bridging the quality chasm. *BMJ* 2001; **323**: 61–62.)

is defined as doing the right things, for the right people, at the right time, and doing them right first time.

FINDING YOUR WAY ROUND THIS BOOK

In this chapter we have looked at the origin and meaning of clinical governance, its relevance to the NHS, and how it is developing. In the next chapter we will look in more detail at some of the models and approaches. In Chapter 3 we will explore the core values of medicine, and what clinical governance will mean for each of us as doctors. Gathering, assessing and using evidence to support the clinical care of patients will be explored in Chapter 4. The need to continually keep up to date through lifelong learning will be emphasized in Chapter 5. In future the performance of doctors (and other health professionals) will be monitored, and approaches used will be set out in Chapter 6. Various aspects of the design, production and use of clinical guidelines are dealt with in Chapter 7. Communication and the documentation of clinical information is explored in Chapter 8, while Chapter 9 looks at the role of health outcomes for monitoring performance. Chapter 10 looks at ideas about teamwork and partnerships with patients, whilst how to work with managers is set out in Chapter 11. Some sources of further information and advice are provided, and there are some ideas and guidance for further reading and references.

Conclusion

The Bristol report paints a clear picture of what is needed for the NHS. 'The culture of the future must be a culture of safety and of quality; a culture of openness and accountability; a culture of public service; a culture in which collaborative teamwork is prized; and a culture of flexibility in which innovation can flourish in response to patients' needs. This book is a contribution to the development of that culture.

REFERENCES

1. Department of Health. *A First Class Service: Quality in the New NHS*. Health Service Circular: HSC(98)113. London: Department of Health, 1998.
2. Coke R. Of the foundation, erection and governance of hospitals. In: *The Shorter Oxford English Dictionary*. Oxford: Oxford University Press, 1992.
3. Public Inquiry into Children's Heart Surgery at the Bristol Royal Infirmary 1984–1995. *Learning from Bristol*. London: Stationery Office, 2001 (Cmnd 5207).
4. Donabedian A. Evaluating the quality of medical care. Milbank *Memorial Fund Quarterly* 1966; **4**: 166–206.
5. Devlin HB. Audit and the quality of clinical care. *Ann R Coll Surg* 1990; **72** (Suppl): 3–14.
6. Maxwell RJ. Quality assessment in health. BMJ 1984; **288**: 1470–1472.
7. World Health Organization, Regional office for Europe. *Targets for Health for All*. Copenhagen: WHO, 1985.
8. WHO Working Group. The principles of quality assurance. *Quality Assurance in Health Care* 1989; **1**: 79–95.
9. Bloor K, Maynard A. *Clinical Governance: Clinician, Heal Thyself?* London: Institute of Health Services Management, 1998.
10. Scally G, Donaldson LJ. Clinical governance and the drive for quality improvement in the new NHS in England. *BMJ* 1998; **317**: 61–65.
11. Bevan G, Bawden D. Clinical data and information, and clinical governance. *Clinical Governance Bulletin* 2001; **2**: 2–3.
12. Committee on Quality of Health Care in America. Crossing the quality chasm: a new health system for the 21st century. Washington, DC: National Academy Press, 2001. In: Kelly MA, Tucci JM. Bridging the quality chasm. *BMJ* 2001; **323**: 61–62.

Clinical governance: principles into practice

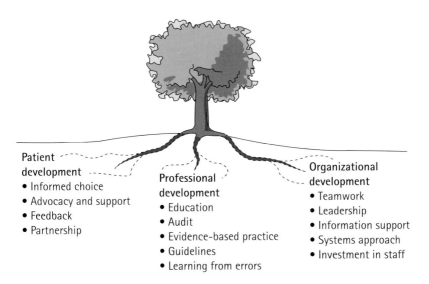

2

There are no simple recipes for clinical governance – good quality care depends on patient, professional and organizational development (Figure 2.1). Efforts to improve care that concentrate on one aspect of development to the neglect of others will underachieve. Similarly there are no easy to assemble models of clinical governance; however, this chapter describes one possible model of clinical governance and attempts to provide some practical guidance on what might help and might hinder its introduction and development. The following areas are covered:

- Structure of clinical governance in an organization and roles of individuals
- Underlying principles of clinical governance
- Quality improvement programmes.

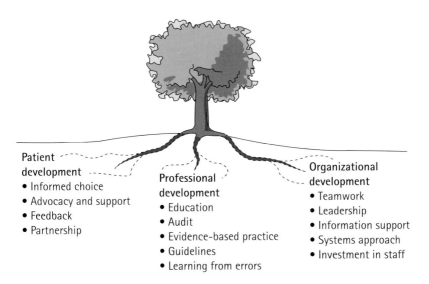

Patient development
- Informed choice
- Advocacy and support
- Feedback
- Partnership

Professional development
- Education
- Audit
- Evidence-based practice
- Guidelines
- Learning from errors

Organizational development
- Teamwork
- Leadership
- Information support
- Systems approach
- Investment in staff

Fig. 2.1 The roots of quality care in health organizations.

STRUCTURE AND ROLES

Hospital or Trust

Clinical governance places a statutory responsibility for ensuring quality health care on the *chief executives* of hospitals and primary care trusts. Previously they have only been judged on how they balance the books. Clinical governance puts the emphasis back on the real priority – patient care. So now the chief executive carries ultimate responsibility for assuring quality in his or her organization, and may be the one in court if things go wrong – a powerful incentive for preventative action.

One of the first tasks for chief executives is the establishment of a sub-committee of the Trust Board to oversee clinical governance in the Trust. Previously the main Board subcommittee was for financial audit, again giving the wrong signals about what was most important in the health service. The Board subcommittee is important as it promotes involvement of *non-executive directors* – these are representatives of the local community who are independent of the Trust and therefore have a key role in overseeing quality within the organization and acting as a 'safe pair of ears'. Their role is to probe and challenge standards of care in the organization as well as motivate and encourage high standards.

The Board subcommittee roles include:

- giving strategic direction and support for clinical governance arrangements in the Trust
- ensuring effective integration with other Trust priorities
- providing a supportive and objective forum for discussion on potentially sensitive and confidential issues of performance within the Trust
- approving clinical governance development plans and receiving regular reports of action plans to ensure that progress is being made
- receiving and reviewing the annual reports on clinical governance from clinical departments in the Trust and providing an independent forum for discussion and review of these reports
- reviewing the effectiveness of response to recommendations from external auditors and assessors, notably the Commission for Health Audit and Inspection.

Membership should include the chief executive, non-executive directors and senior clinicians.

The involvement and commitment of the chief executive sends an important signal to clinical staff about how seriously the hospital or primary care trust takes quality. However, clinical governance is about clinical practice and so it must be led by a clinician. In many hospitals the *clinical governance lead* tends to be the medical director, but it can be the chief nurse or other senior clinician. The clinical governance lead is responsible for co-ordinating and monitoring arrangements, supporting departmental clinical governance leads and reviewing their progress against objectives. They will form a multi-disciplinary team of clinicians to:

- Monitor and promote the ongoing development of clinical governance within the Trust.

- Ensure multidisciplinary working in addressing the clinical governance agenda.
- Co-ordinate and prioritize support for clinical governance leads and departments.
- Review external guidance and identify required action.
- Develop strategies for monitoring performance and assessing progress.

Whereas the subcommittee of the board is responsible for the more strategic development of clinical governance, this clinical governance *steering* or *monitoring group* will be responsible for the day-to-day development and support for clinical governance in departments. Membership should include representatives of departmental clinical governance leads (perhaps on a rotating or rolling annual basis to encourage ownership and new ideas), the organizational leads for education, risk management and information services.

The leadership provided by the chief executive, clinical governance lead and the clinical governance committee is an essential component of the development of clinical governance. Rather than the old-fashioned transactional type of leadership – which relied on hierarchical systems and structures, and reactive organizing and planning – transformational leadership should be the norm. This emphasizes empowerment of staff – leading people to lead themselves – with vision, inspiration and energy rather than authority and control.

An example of a structure for clinical governance in a hospital is shown in Figure 2.2, with the important internal and external influences. In primary

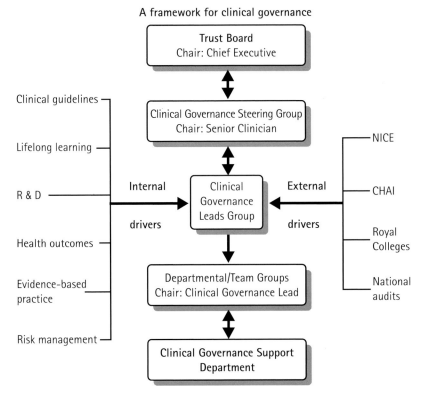

A framework for clinical governance

Fig. 2.2 Organization structure.

care trusts, the more fragmented nature of geographically and historically iso-lated practices creates different problems. Figure 2.3 illustrates the complex-ity of the relationships between individuals and organizations that can exist in developing a structure for quality improvement in a primary care trust.

Department or practice

No amount of committees is going to make clinical governance happen in practice without the real involvement of clinicians on the ward or in the clinic. While the board subcommittee and steering/monitoring group can provide direction and support, it is up to individual departments to deliver the best care for patients. Each department or practice should have a specified *clinical governance lead*. The roles and responsibilities of this lead include:

- Assessing the capability and capacity within the department.
- Identifying weaknesses and deficits in current services.
- Ensuring integration of different quality initiatives and systems within the department (see Box 2.1).
- Producing the annual departmental development plan linked to specific objectives.
- Organizing and chairing departmental meetings.
- Ensuring effective communication and dissemination of information about clinical governance activities both within and between departments.
- Promoting wide multidisciplinary involvement and identifying training and development needs of staff.

Box 2.1   Examples of clinical governance activities

Gastroenterology	– Rolling audit programme of management of patients with GI bleeding, undergoing colonoscopy and having TPN
	– Evidence-based guidelines for endoscopy and upper GI cancers developed and implemented in primary care
	– Risk incidents agreed, collated and fed back on a monthly basis
Surgery	– Establishment of POSSUM scoring system to assess outcomes to co-morbidity of patients
	– Regular view of all CEPOD deaths and lessons discussed
	– Patient focus groups run and user representatives identified for cancer groups
Paediatrics	– Education workshops and ongoing audit about drug errors
	– Learning points from complaints with regular review
	– Care pathways developed for common admissions
	– Audit of communication and subsequent training programme
Obstetrics and gynaecology	– Benchmarking of audit standards with regional hospitals
	– Review and improvement of patient information with Internet access
	– Systematic approach to CPD and staff development initiated
	– Clearer consent guidance for junior staff

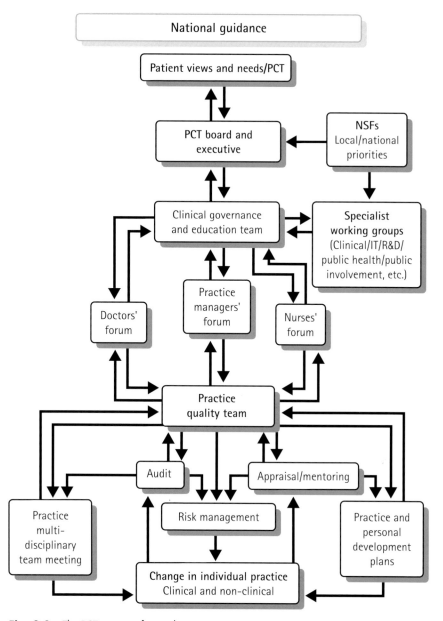

Fig. 2.3 The PCT structure for quality improvement.

Regular meetings of all the departmental clinical governance leads can provide a forum for sharing lessons and improving inter-departmental communication. These meetings can also be used for training and development as regards particular topics.

PRINCIPLES OF CLINICAL GOVERNANCE

Many doctors are cynical about imposed change. The NHS is governed by too many unwritten rules that encourage the status quo (Box 2.2). New ideas about organizational change (such as NHS reforms) or quality improvement (such as clinical audit) have often fallen upon stony ground. However, few health professionals would disagree with the core aim of clinical governance in raising the quality of health care for patients. This is something we all want and something we all know can be improved both in our own clinical practice and that of our colleagues.

Rather than concentrating on how we can ignore the ideas behind clinical governance, we should welcome the opportunity to reduce unacceptable variations in clinical practice, improve quality and attempt to pull together the disparate strands of quality improvement (education, audit, risk management, evidence-based practice, guidelines) and connect the results of these to the planning of future services. The vast majority of doctors genuinely strive to deliver high quality services, and many health professionals have been 'doing' clinical governance for years, albeit in a rather fragmented, haphazard and introspective manner. Clinical governance is an evolutionary development rather than a revolutionary change. Its challenge is for clinicians to be more systematic and open about their quality assurance and harness the energy of the organization to support them.

The Institute of Medicine in the USA has proposed 10 basic rules for changing health services and improving quality of care for patients[4] (Box 2.3). For clinical governance to support the application of these rules, a few underlying principles must be in place: clinical governance should be mainstream; there should be effective teamwork and leadership; collaboration and partnership are pre-requisites; monitoring of progress should be routine and available resources must be used to maximum effect.

Box 2.2   Unwritten rules in the NHS

- We know best
- My own work has no effect on other areas of the NHS
- Clinicians don't need managers
- The more senior you are the more you know!
- Don't admit to mistakes
- Even though we talk about quality we only assess on the quantity
- But I've always done it this way
- There are no rewards for doing well
- Everyone understands the jargon
- It is wrong to seek answers/consult others
- Don't fix it if it's not bust
- Doctors' time is more valuable than nurses'
- Nothing ever changes
- Everything is changing all the time
- The past was much better

(Adapted from: Cullen et al. *British Journal of Clinical Governance* 2000; **5**(4): 233–239.)

Box 2.3   Basic rules for changing health services and improving quality of care[4]

1. *Care based on continuous healing relationships.* Patients should receive care whenever they need it and in many forms, not just face-to-face visits. This rule implies that the health care system should be responsive at all times (24 hours a day, every day) and that access to care should be provided over the Internet, by telephone, and by other means in addition to face-to-face visits.
2. *Customization based on patient needs and values.* The system of care should be designed to meet the most common types of needs, but have the capability to respond to individual patient choices and preferences.
3. *The patient as the source of control.* Patients should be given the necessary information and the opportunity to exercise the degree of control they choose over health care decisions that affect them. The health system should be able to accommodate differences in patient preferences and encourage shared decision making.
4. *Shared knowledge and the free flow of information.* Patients should have unfettered access to their own medical information and to clinical knowledge. Clinicians and patients should communicate effectively and share information.
5. *Evidence-based decision making.* Patients should receive care based on the best available scientific knowledge. Care should not vary illogically from clinician to clinician or from place to place.
6. *Safety as a system property.* Patients should be safe from injury caused by the care system. Reducing risk and ensuring safety require greater attention to systems that help prevent and mitigate errors.
7. *The need for transparency.* The health care system should make information available to patients and their families that allows them to make informed decisions when selecting a health plan, hospital or clinical practice, or choosing among alternative treatments. This should include information describing the system's performance on safety, evidence-based practice and patient satisfaction.
8. *Anticipation of needs.* The health system should anticipate patient needs, rather than simply reacting to events.
9. *Continuous decrease in waste.* The health system should not waste resources or patient time.
10. *Co-operation among clinicians.* Clinicians and institutions should actively collaborate and communicate to ensure an appropriate exchange of information and co-ordination of care.

(Adapted from: Institute of Medicine *Crossing the Quality Chasm.* Washington: National Academy Press, 2001.)

KEEP IT MAINSTREAM

Clinical governance must be part of the main business of health care organizations. The principles of improving the quality of services and providing excellence in clinical care are not optional add-ons. It should be integral to everyday clinical practice for all health professionals. Care should be taken that clinical governance does not become a whole new bureaucracy or side-lined as a discrete activity for a few nominated clinical leads as clinical audit has been in the past. It should become a standing item on all future board, management, policy and divisional meetings rather than exist in a parallel universe. Governance should be as central to Drugs and Therapeutics Committees (through evidence-based decision making and effective monitoring of safe prescribing), or to local Continuing Professional Development groups (through ensuring educational approaches to address quality issues), as it is to audit or quality assurance groups.

Clinical governance is the responsibility of clinicians; however, strong leadership, commitment and direction are needed from senior managers. They will need to ensure that the outcomes of clinical governance effect required change in the planning and development of the organization. Clinical governance should provide the opportunity to reflect on the quality of the organization as well as individual clinicians, and organizational audits such as Investors in People can provide useful standards.

WORK AS TEAMS

One of the problems of audit was that it began as a medical activity and later attempts to tag on multidisciplinary involvement were often unsuccessful. Clinical governance must be a truly multidisciplinary activity. This is not because of political correctness, but because we no longer work as isolated or omniscient individuals. The quality of care a patient receives depends on the care of a whole chain of people, and doctors are just one link in that chain. It is often other health professionals in the chain who are in the best position to identify and correct poor practice, although they have no forum to discuss how improvements can be made.

As the General Medical Council has stressed in their guide on good medical practice, good teamwork is a prerequisite for good medical practice and attention should be paid to how to achieve this. It provides the foundation for reducing inconsistent practice ('He's Dr Jones' patient so we have a different protocol') and for increasing systematic professional development. Teams may exist within departments, such as urology or obstetrics, or may more naturally form between specialties such as Calman cancer groups. However, general medical or surgical responsibilities may lead to joint commitments for delivering the objectives of clinical governance.

Multidisciplinary collaboration within a team is important, but interdisciplinary collaboration between teams should also be promoted. Different clinical teams treating the same clinical conditions or the same patients can exist in different compartments, with little communication and considerable variation in practice. In hospitals, nursing staff who accompany medical staff on their separate ward rounds will testify to the problems of juggling different decisions made on the same patient. Often neglected groups such as out-of-hours staff should be involved.

DEVELOP EFFECTIVE LEADERSHIP

Joint medical and nursing clinical governance leads should be established to promote a multidisciplinary approach. The clinical governance leads for each department or team must be people who have the confidence of their colleagues and the leadership potential to provide direction and encourage effective change. The leads will be responsible for organizing and chairing meetings, setting agendas, ensuring attendance and reporting back to the main clinical governance group. They should be encouraged to develop formal (learning sets, peer review groups) or informal links with colleagues in other hospitals or primary care groups to share ideas and promote development. Good leaders will challenge the status quo and provide direction for improving systems of care.

Although there will be a natural tendency to reflect medical dominance in the composition of clinical governance groups, responsibility should be shared within teams or departments to gain wider involvement. Different roles, such as education, audit, risk management, R&D or communication can be assigned to different clinical leads from different clinical disciplines – this encourages a *portfolio* approach with different staff in the department rotating between lead roles and responsibilities. This will also encourage wider ownership and understanding about quality issues.

Enthusiasm should be an essential selection criterion for these clinical governance leads. The Director of Human Resources in hospitals or primary care trusts will have an important role in supporting the training and development of new skills in leadership and facilitation. Contributions should be recognized, valued and rewarded. Incentives such as promotion, resource allocation, development funding and merit awards should be agreed. Sanctions should not be overplayed as this will alienate rather than involve people. Win the sceptics and the doubters over with successes.

COLLABORATE

Greater attention must be paid to encouraging closer involvement of patients and to linking primary and secondary care. Quality should be viewed from a patient's perspective and not as separate compartments for separate destinations on the patient's health service journey. Efforts should be made to incorporate what patients value (for example, accessibility, information and communication, interpersonal skills) as well as more technical professional values for quality of care. Patient involvement may be easier to obtain in primary care settings than secondary care where contact is often brief and irregular. Advice from general advocacy groups such as Patient Advice and Liaison Service (PALS) or Patient Forums, or specific groups such as the Stroke Association or cancer support groups may provide a starting point.

The quality of health care, whether a well-managed discharge of a patient from hospital to the required supportive environment, or the appropriateness of an emergency admission to hospital, requires excellent communication between health professionals. Communication can be strengthened through specific district meetings, such as agreeing guidelines for best practice and referral, or through more innovative steps such as developing e-mail access between general practitioners and hospital specialists to discuss individual patients.

Greater collaboration with patients and external stakeholders such as primary or secondary care trusts also provides valuable feedback on progress from outside the organization. It is easy for staff in a hospital or practice to become complacent and believe that everything is going swimmingly. Getting the views of service users and those outside the hospital or practice can provide a more objective and informative appraisal of standards of care inside.

MONITOR PROGRESS

One of the key principles behind clinical governance is that it should be a bottom-up initiative. Any authoritarian approach will not only lead to dissonance, but will be unenforceable, as trying to police so many different teams and professionals would require huge resources. However, progress will need to be monitored, and this can be considered at both departmental or team level, and at individual level.

Each department or team should have its own objectives and annual plan which will form the basis of review and evaluation of progress. In order to make improvements, each team must be clear about what it is trying to accomplish, how this will be implemented and how they will be able to demonstrate change. So objectives should be SMART (specific, measurable, achievable, realistic and timely). The more specific the objective, the more likely it is that improvement will occur.

Lead responsibilities, outcomes and timescales should be explicit. Each departmental report should be concise and follow a consistent framework to avoid the tendency of everyone sending in reams of uninformative details. A starting point for each department or team should be to reflect on examples of what has worked well in the past and why.

Priority topics for clinical governance may be obvious from team discussions; however, there may also be considerable differences in opinions. One way of deciding is by voting for topic areas. This way every member of a team has a chance to influence the final choice rather than just one or two senior medical staff deciding. Keeping the voting secret will prevent any potential for intimidation or suppression of views.

At an individual level, clinical governance must be a central part of staff appraisal and performance review. Obligations should be made explicit in contracts for future appointments and should be integrated into job plans for current staff. Appraisal of doctors will be an integral part of clinical governance, and training may be required for both appraisers and appraisees.

The initial emphasis of clinical governance should be on establishing systems for positive quality improvement rather than the more threatening and difficult issues around searching for medical failure (Box 2.4). However, tackling poor performance by developing systems of early recognition, regular appraisal and support will be needed (see Chapter 6).

RESOURCES

Efficient use of existing resources is important. Within the limitations of existing resources each team or department will need to review what support is

---

Box 2.4   Steps for developing clinical governance

1. Each department should hold a time out to discuss the implications of clinical governance. This should be chaired by the lead clinician and involve all senior staff. The following questions should be considered:

   - *What is the situation now in the department? What examples are there of good practice and what examples are there of poor practice?*
   - *What are the areas for improvement within existing resources? How can such improvement be achieved?*
   - *What structure and what realistic support (staff, IT, library, training, etc.) does each department need for clinical governance?*
   - *How can effective multidisciplinary involvement be achieved?*

2. Nursing and medical clinical governance leads should be chosen from each department.
3. The timing and content of clinical governance meetings should be agreed. Dedicated roles should be assigned to different clinicians to ensure shared responsibility for progress.
4. Each department should develop their own programme which includes clear objectives and targets for review that reflect local priorities.
5. Departmental programmes should be reviewed by a steering group. The key principle for clinical governance should be self-regulation but with a strong emphasis on transparency and clear reporting.
6. Training and development needs for leadership and specific skills within each department should be identified.
7. A monthly Trust Clinical Governance group comprising the clinical governance leads from all departments should be established.
8. Steps should be taken to establish or strengthen a district-wide forum for clinical governance leads from Trusts, primary care groups and the health authority.

---

required and what skills are necessary to deliver their agenda of clinical governance. There are four key areas of resources to be considered:

1. STAFF There are staff in a number of areas who will have important roles to play in supporting clinical governance. These include audit or clinical governance support departments; risk management; complaints and litigation; information services and coding; library; education and training. Clinical governance support department staff should move away from conducting small, project-based audits. They have a central co-ordinating role in supporting clinical governance groups as well as collecting and collating the information which will drive change (Box 2.5, Figure 2.4). The skill mix of these staff should be reviewed regularly to ensure that they meet the future needs of clinical governance groups.

2. TIME The lack of time in today's over-stretched NHS is a major hurdle to achieving success. If clinical governance and teamworking are to be taken seriously then protected time must be committed. Review the time committed to clinical duties, administrative and managerial responsibilities, teaching, research and professional development. Effective time management is essential. There may be a plethora of groups covering these aspects which can be reviewed and rationalized. Hospital doctors have the advantage over other health professionals in

Clinical governance: principles into practice

Box 2.5   Sources of information and drivers of change: a foundation for review and reporting by teams and departments

- **Lifelong learning, education and training** – identification of individual and team needs; planning of personal development programmes with local colleagues; reflection of methods used and preferred methods of learning.
- **Clinical risk management** – regular critical/untoward incident reporting; monthly examples of an adverse incident from which lessons can be learnt; review of procedures and systems to reduce risks identified. This information should be used for learning and not for blame.
- **Audit** – identification of key audit areas (e.g. national audits and confidential enquiries); feedback of individualized data; establishment of sustainable and continuous audits in key chosen areas.
- **Evidence-based practice** – dissemination and action on key reviews (e.g. Effective Health Care Bulletins); access and use of sources of evidence (Cochrane Library and Clinical Evidence).
- **Clinical guidelines** – development or adaptation (e.g. from NICE) of guidelines that are based on evidence rather than anecdote and then effective implementation.
- **Complaints and litigation** – reviewing numbers and types of cases and ensuring regular feedback and discussion within individual teams.
- **Communication and record-keeping** – improving documentation of care and standards of communication across the Trust.
- **R&D** – local research projects; dissemination of innovative practice; getting research into practice.
- **Health outcomes** – clinical indicators (e.g. mortality after MI or surgery) and clinical effectiveness indicators (e.g. CABG or hip replacement rates); development of outcomes that will reflect quality of care and can be used to inform clinical practice.
- **Multidisciplinary and inter-agency working** – collaboration with primary care trusts and the health authority; strengthening of teamworking.
- **Patient involvement** – approaches to obtain patient views and incorporation of these into future practice on an ongoing basis. This will require active participation of patients and carers in clinical governance groups.
- **Staff appraisal** – linking governance objectives with staff appraisal.

These components should be coherent rather than being separate pieces of a jigsaw (see Figure 2.4). For example, review of complaints or critical incidents should prompt a review of current practice, the development of evidence-based guidelines and training programmes to improve practice.

having protected time for clinical governance and education and this time must be used effectively. Clinical governance should be seen as an opportunity for allocating protected time for other health professionals. In primary care steps should be taken to provide cover for meetings. Individual practices could be covered by neighbouring practices. Deputizing services may be able to provide cover for groups of practices to hold joint meetings.

Improving quality is not something to be done on the third Tuesday lunchtime of every month. However, protected time of about one session a week should be allocated for clinical governance leads to recognize the commitment involved. Protected time should also be agreed for departmental or team meetings during one session each month. It may be that there is some knock-on effect on waiting times or activity, but this may be the cost of ensuring a quality service.

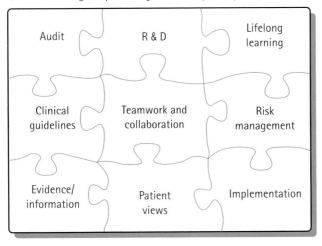

Fig. 2.4 The jigsaw model.

3. INFORMATION TECHNOLOGY Investment in information systems is crucial if clinical governance is to work properly. Today's dependence on laborious and unrewarding case note review and data collection is not sustainable. Fully integrated patient management systems already exist in many general practices and are being introduced in most hospitals in the near future. This opportunity should be seized. At present there is much routine information entered onto computer databases which could be used to greater effect. Work should begin in improving the consistency and validity of recording and coding of this information. Key indicators should be agreed by individual teams and departments for regular feedback of performance. These could be quality indicators such as the wound infection rate or appropriateness indicators such as the proportion of patients who go on to revascularization after angiography.

Information technology also has an important role in improving access to clinical information. Knowledge databases such as Medline and the Cochrane Library can be networked to wards and clinic rooms. Clinical evidence should be available where and when decisions are being taken about patient care and not imprisoned in distant libraries.

4. TRAINING There is considerable ignorance and uncertainty about what clinical governance involves. Much effort is required to raise awareness and understanding. Departmental time outs will provide the first steps for achieving this as well as promoting wider debate and team building. Specific skills such as teaching, mentoring, negotiation, IT, critical appraisal skills or measuring health outcomes may be identified with time. Regional and national initiatives should provide some support in training and awareness. Local expertise should also be identified.

One of the problems as regards historical allocation of resources is that it has often gone to pet projects or to the clinicians who shout loudest. Clinical governance provides an opportunity to ensure equitable distribution of resources. The senior clinical governance lead in the organization will be in a position of authority to ensure that this happens in line with local and national priorities. This strategic overview will also enable greater efforts to be made to involve patients in deciding what areas of clinical care can be improved and to promote collaboration between primary and secondary care.

One opportunity for clinical governance is to be more innovative and systematic in our approach to implementing change. Much activity has been dissipated in the past in conducting audits to show inappropriate X-ray requests or laboratory and pathology requests with little effort put into promoting change. A 15-minute outreach visit to a GP or hospital doctor may be a worthwhile investment if it improves the appropriateness of requests. Likewise a consensus meeting to agree local clinical practice guidelines may improve standards of care and free up time by reducing inappropriate referrals (see Figure 2.3).

PROGRAMMES TO IMPROVE QUALITY

There are no simple recipes for achieving successful clinical governance programmes. Some will work, raising the standards of care for patients and the self-esteem of professionals. Others will splutter and die, leaving only a ghost to nag. Hindsight is a great teacher and a review of the research literature about what distinguishes the successes from the failures can help to inform us about the essential components of a good quality programme (Box 2.6).

The use of a framework for clinical governance projects can be valuable. We have a structure for taking clinical histories and conducting clinical examinations, to remind us how to be thorough and systematic. Similarly, a structure or model for undertaking clinical governance work can help us to be thorough and systematic, and provides an explicit guide for all staff to understand and to follow.

REVIEW, AGREE, IMPLEMENT AND DEMONSTRATE (RAID)

The Clinical Governance Support Team uses the *review, agree, implement and demonstrate* (RAID) model for development of delegates from participating organizations (Figure 2.5). The aim is to challenge mindsets and traditional practices, and help staff to define new and innovative ways of delivering the best care for patients.

The review process is based on a number of key components:

1. Multidisciplinary workshops to allow all staff to explore how to improve services.
2. Involvement and discussions with all staff involved in the patient pathway of care, including the patients themselves.
3. Establishing current performance through information such as waiting times, activity, patient satisfaction, costs.

2

Box 2.6 **Essential criteria for a successful quality programme**

- Recognize and build on existing effective quality activities.
- Enable professionals and managers to work together to improve quality, to be clear about their different responsibilities and to build mutual understanding, trust and respect.
- Build on and extend professionals' skills, in a way that they believe will help them in their everyday work and careers.
- Provide training in quality methods at the time when people need the skills in their quality activities and projects.
- Give training and learning materials which do not introduce unnecessarily complicated concepts and 'jargon', use examples from a relevant professional service and a variety of learning methods to develop the new competencies which are required.
- Combine both profession-specific and multidisciplinary training and projects.
- Ensure projects are managed and work on organizationally important and authorized problems, follow a structured approach, and make real changes which achieve measured improvements.
- Allow flexibility for different parts of the organization to use effective methods which are appropriate to their activities.
- Provide an over-arching coherence which avoids different 'quality language' and which also co-ordinates different activities.
- Energize and realize people's untapped potential, and provide a way to fulfil values and to gain a greater satisfaction from work and serving others.

(Adapted from John Ovreveit, Norwegian Medical Association, 1999.)

RAID model

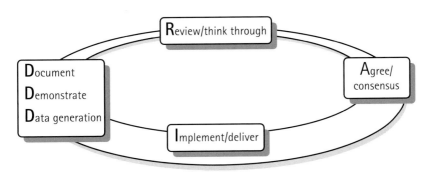

Fig. 2.5 The RAID model.

4. Review of documentation to assess how the programme of work fits in with local and national priorities.
5. Mapping of the patient pathway to provide an overview of the process of care and allow insight into what it is like to be a patient.

A summary of the review process and subsequent recommendations is then written up to describe the evidence for 'where we are now' and the challenges of 'where we want to be'.

The review process is a fundamental part of gaining agreement. Agreement is a gradual process that starts with the raising of awareness and understanding, and ends with ownership and commitment. Ideas that are identified for improvement can then be adopted and implemented (see Chapter 7), starting with projects that will provide quick wins and demonstrate early results in improving quality of care.

Demonstration of change is an essential part of quality improvement. It allows staff to evaluate and reflect on their performance. It also promotes expertise in and ownership of health information and can prompt review of what measures are important to collect. Information such as health outcomes, clinical indicators, access times, costs, activity and diagnostic test requests can be used over time to monitor change, or in comparison with other organizations to benchmark performance (see Chapter 9).

PLAN, DO, STUDY, ACT (PDSA)

The RAID model used by the Clinical Governance Support Team is based on the quality cycle first proposed by Deming in the 1950s as a systematic approach for businesses to adopt to continuously improve and respond to customers' needs. The *Plan, Do, Study and Act* (PDSA) model (Figure 2.6) has been adopted by 'collaborative' networks in UK and US health services and involves a cycle of review and planning for improvements (Plan); implementation of small changes (Do); monitoring change through agreed measures (Study) and implementing further change on the basis of early results (Act).

The aim of the model is to encourage constant change, reflection and demonstrable improvement. It recognizes the dynamic nature of quality improvement, and how we learn from experience and feedback. Most im-

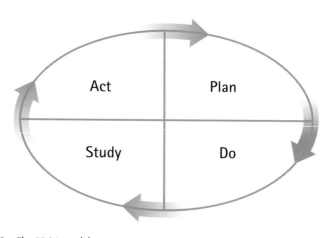

Fig. 2.6 The PDSA model.

Clinical governance: principles into practice

portantly it is a quick and simple model for testing new ideas to improve quality of care. The PDSA cycle provides an achievable stepwise approach to change:

- *PLAN* – plan the change you intend to introduce to improve patient care. Clarify the aims of the planned change and how you will measure the change. Agree the information necessary to demonstrate change (e.g. waiting times, proportion of patients on an appropriate drug, numbers of drug errors) and the timescale for measurement of this information. Start with small ideas, but if the planned change is complex, then break it down into bite-size chunks.
- *DO* – put the change into practice and measure its impact by collecting the agreed data. Keep this step as short as possible and identify any problems or barriers along the way.
- *STUDY* – review and analyse the data. Has there been change? Could things have been done better?
- *ACT* – change the plan to focus on what works and change what did not work. Go back to the 'DO' step and measure further change.

Both the RAID and the PDSA models provide an easy mnemonic for thinking about, implementing and evaluating change in real practice settings. They emphasize that quality improvement is a continuous evolution of small changes rather than a big bang that is too ambitious to ever take place. The cycles of change are small but clever adaptations that can happen tomorrow afternoon rather than large trials that will take years to start. Problems can be quickly identified and changed rather than wasting time waiting for long-term outcomes.

FURTHER READING

Berwick DM. A primer on leading the improvement of systems. *BMJ* 1996; **312**: 619.

General Medical Council. *Good Medical Practice: Guidance from the General Medical Council.* London: GMC, 1995.

Secretary of State for Health. *A First Class Service: Quality in the NHS.* London: Stationery Office, 1998.

Core values in medicine

'Life is not really the most important thing in life. Some cling to it as a miser to his money, and to as little purpose. Others wear it lightly – ready to risk it for a cause, a hope, a song, the wind on their face.'

Sir Theodore Fox: Lancet, 1965

In this chapter we look at:

- The consultation as the central task of medicine
- Professionalism
- The role of the doctor
- The doctor–patient relationship
- Values.

THE CONSULTATION – THE CENTRAL TASK OF MEDICINE

'The essential unit of medical practice is the occasion when in the intimacy of the consulting room or the sick room, a person who is ill, or believes himself to be ill, seeks the advice of a doctor whom he trusts. This is a consultation and all else in medicine derives from it.' So wrote Sir James Spence some 40 years ago.[1]

The consultation is therefore the central task of medicine, and confidence of the patient in the doctor is at the heart of the doctor–patient relationship.[2]

PROFESSIONALISM

Medical professionalism has been described as resting on three pillars which together constitute the basis of doctors' independence and their autonomy; expertise, ethics and service[3] (Figure 3.1).

Expertise derives from the body of knowledge and skills whose utility is constantly invigorated by the results of research. From the time of the Hippocratic oath medical practice has always had a very strong ethical foundation. Ethical behaviour derives from a combination of values and standards, while service embodies a vocational commitment to put patients first.

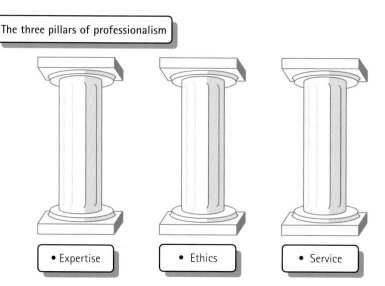

The three pillars of professionalism

- Expertise   - Ethics   - Service

Fig. 3.1 The three pillars of medical professionalism. (Adapted from: Irvine DH. The performance of doctors. I. Professionalism and self regulation in a changing world. *BMJ* 1997; **314**: 1540–1542.)

THE ROLE OF THE DOCTOR

From a different perspective, the sociologist, Talcot Parsons, in describing theoretical aspects of the doctor's role, lists three: technical competence, emotional neutrality and orientation towards others.[4] Stereotypical doctors, such as the medical characters in television soap operas or classic books such as A.J. Cronin's *Dr Finlay's Casebook*, are portrayed as displaying the highest technological skill, whilst remaining aloof.

More recently the doctor's roles have been defined as providing high quality care, through being concerned with diagnosis, prognosis, treatment and the planning of care, with communication of this to the patient; a concern not only with the individual but with the community; and managing resources effectively, including skills, time, facilities and finance. This can be combined with a view from the perspective of the patient (Box 3.1).[5]

Box 3.1 The patient perspective in clinical practice

What is wrong with me?   Diagnosis
What does this mean for me?   Prognosis
What can be done for me?   Treatment and care
What can I learn from this patient?   Research
What can others benefit?   The public health dimension
What can I teach others?   Education and training

(After: Calman K. The profession of medicine. *BMJ* 1994; 309: 1140–1143.)

THE DOCTOR–PATIENT RELATIONSHIP

Three models of the doctor–patient 'transactional' relationship have been described (Box 3.2).[6] Firstly, there can be total authority on the part of the doctor and complete submission on the part of the patient. Such a situation is the parent–child relationship and is appropriate when the doctor has to deal with a comatose patient. The second model is that of guidance and co-operation, where the relationship is more like that between a parent and his or her child or adolescent. The doctor is much more powerful than the patient, but has much to offer. This position might occur where the patient is acutely ill, perhaps with an infection such as pneumonia or a surgical emergency such as a perforated bowel. The third role is more akin to that of counsellor. Here the doctor and patient meet as equals, one adult with another. This latter model is the one that fits most closely the experience of the general practitioner and is increasingly sought by patients from all doctors.

Box 3.2   Three models of the doctor–patient relationship

Dominance and submission: total authority of the doctor with complete submission of the patient

Guidance and cooperation: a parent–child relationship

The doctor as counsellor: the doctor and patient are equals

VALUES

In 1995 a national conference considered that the profession's core values included commitment, caring, competence and integrity (Box 3.3).[7]

Commitment

Commitment can be defined as the action of entrusting, or an obligation undertaken. In medicine, the impact of this cannot be underestimated: it is lifelong, and transcends notions of a 'normal job' – it is not 'nine to five'. In general practice this can mean seeing patients over many years. Although less

---

Box 3.3   Core values for medicine

Commitment
Caring
Competence
Integrity
Confidentiality
Ability to work in a team
Concern for the individual and the community
Education and training
Contributing to the knowledge base of the discipline

Box 3.4 Commitment: patients as people (1)

A doctor was running a regular diabetes clinic. With some years of experience he had come to associate a fat stack of notes in young people with poorly controlled diabetes, and regular advice seemingly falling on deaf ears with the patient not understanding, not believing, or just not caring.

One set of notes 8 inches thick were for a young lady who had had diabetes for 20 years. There were numerous entries documenting high blood sugar, poor compliance with attempts to gain better control, a progressive decline in renal function and extensive retinopathy.

Instead of a difficult patient, the doctor was faced with a charming and intelligent young lady. She was fully aware of the implications of poor control, but terrified of hypoglycaemic attacks and the disastrous effect these had on her work. Her attempts to gain better control of her diabetes had resulted in hypoglycaemic episodes early in the morning, and she was under pressure from her manager because of all the time taken off for hospital visits. She did not want to lose her job.

The doctor reflected that she had been asked to aim for a level of control that produced side effects incompatible with her lifestyle. This had led to poor compliance, mutual frustration and distrust between doctor and patient, and the onset of complications.

The doctor now tries to remember that, although doctors are often influenced only by medical factors, patients are pulled in many different directions by social, psychological and medical influences, and they attach different priorities to those of doctors. Failing to account for these differences will inevitably prevent the delivery of effective care.

(Adapted from: Daniels RJ. It is too easy to blame only the patient. *BMJ* 2001; **323**: 31.)

common in hospital practice, many patients do attend regularly or repeatedly over many years (see Box 3.4). It is important that patients are seen as people (see Boxes 3.5 and 3.6).

Box 3.5 Commitment: patients as people (2)

It was a busy Friday night in casualty. One doctor was absent, and there had been a major accident. All the staff had been looking after seriously injured patients for some time; not all of them had survived, and emotions were running high. The backlog of minor injuries had built up to a 6-hour wait, and tempers were fraying in the waiting room.

The doctor returned to start clearing the backlog, but was feeling super-efficient and slightly short tempered, thinking that didn't the patients realize the staff had to deal with far more important things than cut fingers or drunks?

The doctor picked the next card out of the box and went into the cubicle. With barely a glance at the patient she brusquely asked what was the matter. A middle-aged man looked at her and said, nonchalantly, 'I was preparing for my usual Friday night sexual activity when the chandelier broke, and I fell into the vat of custard'.

Looking at him in disbelief, 'Really?' the doctor asked. 'No,' he said, 'but I've been sitting in the waiting room for two hours trying to pluck up the courage to say that'.

The doctor grinned, asked what had really happened, and the patient told her what he had done. The doctor relaxed, treated him and chatted to him as a real person, not just a patient. She spent the rest of the shift smiling.

The doctor was inspired to think that someone faced with a long wait had thought up something like that, and kept it in his mind without getting annoyed or impatient. He changed her perspective, brightened up her evening, and reminded her of the fact that people, not patients, were in the waiting room. The doctor still thinks about him when she is having a bad day.

(Adapted from: Whybrew K. A chandelier and a vat of custard. *BMJ* 2001; **322**: 1480.)

Box 3.6 Commitment: patients as people (3)

One Saturday afternoon while servicing his car, a doctor got a splinter of metal in his index finger which he could not extract. He went to the accident and emergency department, still grubby and oily, where he had trained and worked. On a whim he decided not to say he was a doctor.

He queued at reception and was interrogated: name, address, date of birth, GP's name and address, religion and next of kin. He suggested that, as he was unlikely to die, the receptionist could manage without his religion or next of kin. It was quickly made clear to him that without a religion he would not be seen. Having declared Church of England, he was allowed into the waiting area, and directed to a queue that he guessed to be 'minor ops'. For half an hour little happened. A few more patients joined various queues and a couple of nurses chatted quietly in a corner, but there was no sign of anyone else.

Suddenly the hall was full of chattering medical students and casualty officers. The penny dropped; they had all been watching the men's Wimbledon final on television.

Three of the students worked their way along the now lengthy queue inspecting the various injuries. All three glanced at his card; two of them picked up his finger, examined it briefly, and let it drop into his lap without saying a word or even establishing eye contact.

The doctor patient worked out what was happening. The students were coming to the end of their accident and emergency attachment. They were feeling fairly confident; they had done several ring blocks and were looking for something more interesting.

Eventually a doctor arrived to deal with the student rejects. Quickly and competently he gave the patient a ring block, removed the splinter and dressed the finger.

On reflection, the doctor had been treated, not as a person with a minor injury, but as a supplicant, a fearful child, and the disembodied owner of a rather boring finger. He thought this would never have happened had he announced on arrival that he was a doctor.

(Adapted from: Kendell R. On the receiving end. *BMJ* 2000; **321**: 1067.)

Caring

Caring, and compassion, in doctoring can come in many guises. Sometimes it is just about the doctor being there (see Box 3.7). At other times it can just be about seeing beyond the superficialities, for example, of presenting

Box 3.7 Caring and compassion (1)

The patient had passed from one doctor to another. She was a Yemenite widow aged about 68 who often attended, although she suffered only from abdominal pain. She had countless consultations, visits to emergency departments, ultrasound examinations, endoscopies and barium enemas, but the cause of the pain could not be found. Psychiatric consultations suggested masked depression but were no other help. Medication was ineffective.

After nearly 3 years, the patient attended again, at the end of a busy day and without an appointment. The doctor, out of frustration, thought he would teach her a lesson and let her wait. She finally entered the consulting room, ready for the 'fight' and reinforced by her 54-year-old daughter. She cried and presented with a pain like that of peritonitis.

After clinical examination the doctor asked about the multiple burn scars; he had noticed these before but had had no time to ask about them. They were coin-shaped scars all over her body from scalp to feet. He was told of the traditional Yemenite remedy of branding the skin of the area in pain with a red-hot iron nail, and of children's fears beforehand, blindfolded and with their hands and feet tied. The doctor learned from the daughter of the death of the patient's mother when she was 7 years old and of her move to a Jewish foster home to hide from a Yemeni law of conversion of all orphans to Islam. She had been forced to marry aged 12, still without menses, a mother at 14, and a widow at 16. She married again, to an aged cousin and had another seven children, two of them with Down's syndrome. This second husband became an abusive alcoholic when they moved to Israel. Two of her children were in jail, two in psychiatric institutions, and two were abroad. The only carer was her first daughter, herself married with an alcoholic husband and a mother of a Down's syndrome daughter.

This hour was the turning point for doctor and patient; from now on he considered they were together in no man's land: neither his medicine nor her folk healers could repair her basic mistrust in life and mankind. The doctor was astonished, moved and compassionate for this woman.

Since then she continues to attend, still with abdominal pain and still without appointments, but she no longer asks for further referrals. Sometimes the doctor examines her, sometimes they just talk about her pain. They mainly pass about 10 minutes together in deep respect for her suffering, mourning all her losses and accepting the new role she cast the doctor in: just being there.

(Adapted from: Matalon A. Just being there. *BMJ* 2001; **322**: 342.)

symptoms (see Box 3.8). Without understanding the impact that illness has on a patient's life, it can be difficult to know whether or not the care being provided is doing what was intended to reduce the impact of the disease. Medical systems can inadvertently add to the patient's burden, such as

---

Box 3.8 Caring and compassion (2)

A consultant trainer describes a teaching ward session, and asking a student who she had seen the previous night. 'Nobody exciting – just another chronic chest.'

The student did well, giving a succinct description of the patient's illness, her assessment, the treatment given, and admission to the ward. She demonstrated the physical signs with confidence. Respiratory physiology and pathology were discussed. The consultant got the students to measure peak flow rate, FEV_1 and ventilatory capacity. They went on to discuss gas transfer and respiratory failure, particularly in relation to chronic obstructive bronchitis, emphysema and the hypersecretion of mucus. Risk factors, genetics and the mechanisms of inflammation were covered, before moving on to the use of steroids and long-term oxygen.

The consultant was thumbing through the case notes, and noticed admissions five or six times during the previous year. The story was the same: 'exacerbation of chronic chest disease' in the middle of the night, leading to admission to hospital for 4 or 5 days, with similar treatment on each occasion.

'What about the social history?' asked the consultant. The team listened to the story of a retired labourer who, until 2 years ago, had smoked 20 or more cigarettes a day, who lived alone, whose wife had died, and who had no close relatives.

'But what is his life really like?' The student gently took the patient's hand and asked. He rarely went out of his tiny flat, living on his own with 'meals on wheels' the high point of the day. 'Why did he call the emergency service at 2.00 am?' The student turned back to her patient. He described the limitations imposed by his disease, his lack of involvement with life, his feelings of uselessness. Looking straight at the student he said quietly: 'It's the same every night. I just want to sleep forever'. A tear trickled down his cheek: 'But I am not allowed to ask, am I?'

(Adapted from: Neale G. Just another chronic chest. *BMJ* 2001; **322**: 901.)

Box 3.9   Caring and compassion (3)

In order to understand more clearly the effects that anticoagulant treatment was having on a patient's life, the patient was given a small disposable camera, costing £5–7, and asked to take pictures. When the photographs were developed, the patient and a nurse developed a storyboard of a typical day in the life of a patient taking warfarin.

The photographs added a previously unsuspected dimension for the doctor: the journey to have blood taken, the complications of getting the results, the timing of doses, and more.

The doctor was struck that, although anticoagulant treatment is relatively straightforward, it was having a profound effect on this patient.

What about a person with diabetes, a person with disabilities, or someone undergoing chemotherapy? Here is a new, cheap and simple way to see the world of patients.

Written consent would be needed if the photographs were going to be shown to others.

(Adapted from: Wilson T. A gadget that changed my perspective. *BMJ* 2001; **323**: 845.)

through complicated schedules, e.g. medication, appointments systems, investigations (see Box 3.9).

Competence

People expect their doctors to be knowledgeable and skilled, and trust them to provide the highest standard of care. To achieve this they must be competent and perform consistently well. Whilst this is true for doctors practising in any milieu, there is a particular facet in general practice, where the doctor is faced with a myriad of undifferentiated symptoms, many of which are ultimately trivial or minor. Here the competence and skill are particularly about distinguishing the serious from the trivial (see Box 3.10).

Box 3.10   Competence (1)

It was a busy Saturday morning surgery. The patient was a 52-year-old man the doctor knew vaguely. His partner called at about 10.30 am when there were still 15 patients to see and three visits in the book. The patient had attended the day before with a sore throat and had been given penicillin by another doctor. The partner told the doctor that he was no better and was having difficulty breathing. The GP asked if the man could come to the surgery but was told he found it very difficult to get down the stairs.

The GP spoke directly to the patient. He had a slight sore throat but was not wheezy, and could talk normally without obvious breathing problems. There was no history of asthma or allergy. He felt fine in bed but could not get down stairs and found it an effort to go to the lavatory.

The doctor visited after surgery and found the patient looking fine lying in bed, and conversing easily without dyspnoea or stridor. Impatiently, the doctor asked the patient to sit up so he could look at his throat and examine his chest. 'I can't, Doctor.' 'Of course you can', said the GP firmly helping him upright, at which point he choked and gasped and threw himself back flat on the bed. Trying again, the result was the same. He was unable to breathe in the vertical position but was fine lying flat.

Examination while flat showed a little redness of the pharynx, but no quinsy or obvious swelling, and no cervical glands. He had a slight temperature. The lungs were clear with no abnormality.

When asked about any past problems, he had some polyps removed as a child.

The patient was admitted, with the ambulance crew receiving instructions to keep him lying flat. After 48 hours of steroids and antibiotics, the patient had his posterior laryngeal polyp removed. This had been flopping in and out of the glottic opening as the patient changed position from horizontal to vertical and back again, causing 'iatrogenic' laryngeal obstruction.

(Adapted from: Price J. Not an ordinary sore throat. *BMJ* 2000; **321**: 1264.)

Box 3.11   Competence (2)

The patient, Mr M, was a rather formal gentleman in his early 60s. He developed late onset asthma and regularly attended a major London teaching hospital. He later developed prostatic symptoms, and the general practitioner recommended he should go back to the same hospital, where they had his records, and to a particular urologist to whom the GP usually referred his patients. The patient left to talk things over with his wife.

He returned a few days later, saying that a relative had suggested another urologist in private practice. However, the patient was uncertain about this, and asked the opinion of the GP. The doctor said that the patient had mentioned his confidence in the consultant he had seen for his asthma at the hospital, and his confidence in the hospital, but added that it was the patient's decision. He said he would talk it over with his wife.

On his third visit the patient was still undecided. The doctor rose from his seat and invited the patient to take his chair while he took the patient's seat. Leaning forward, he then said, 'Dr M, you know my problem with the chest, and now the prostate, what do you think I should do?' Without any hesitation Mr M leaned forward, put his hand confidentially on the doctor's knee, and said, 'With this story, I think you should go to the teaching hospital'.

He did so, and had successful surgery. Role reversal is now a useful approach in the GP's armamentarium.

(Adapted from: Law R. Decisions, decisions, decisions .... *BMJ* 2001; **322**: 351.)

Competence among all doctors does not imply uniformity, particularly of style. It can also be advantageous to be able to think and act laterally (see Boxes 3.9 and 3.11).

Confidentiality

Confidentiality must be a core value for medicine. According to the Declaration of Geneva of 1948, the doctor must respect the secrets that are confided by patients. There is no doubt that a doctor owes a duty of confidentiality to those who consult him or her. It is generally held that this duty even extends after the death of the patient. However, this duty is not absolute and there are a number of exceptions, but the doctor must always be prepared to justify actions.

If the patient gives proper consent, then, of course, the doctor is free to make disclosure. The doctor in Britain is obliged to disclose information on the order of a court. There is a statutory duty under certain public health regulations to notify certain infectious diseases.

> **Box 3.12 Advice and treatment for those aged under 16 years of age**
>
> A Mrs Gillick, who had five daughters, sought an assurance from her local health authority that they would not give advice and treatment concerning contraception to her daughters whilst they were under the age of 16 without her prior knowledge and consent. Failing to receive such an assurance she applied to the court for a declaration that the health authority could not lawfully give such advice or treatment as this was against the law relating to parental rights. The case eventually reached the House of Lords where the decision was that parental rights were recognized by law only as long as they were needed for the protection of the child, and such rights were yielded to the child's rights to his or her own decisions when they were of sufficient understanding and intelligence as to be capable of making up their own mind. This means that a girl under 16 can give consent for contraceptive advice and treatment by a doctor. The doctor has a discretion to give contraceptive advice and treatment without the parents' knowledge provided the doctor is satisfied that she has a sufficient understanding and intelligence to appreciate fully what is proposed. This fact must apply in each case.
>
> (Gillick v West Norfolk and Wisbech Area Health Authority and the DHSS (1985) 3 WLR 830 3 AER 402)

There can be particular circumstances where a doctor believes it to be necessary to sometimes give information in confidence to a close relative without formally seeking the patient's consent. However, there is a particular situation with regard to children under the age of 16 years, following a much publicized court case (see Box 3.12).

Confidentiality can be threatened in ways that it may be difficult to imagine (see Box 3.13). The doctor in this anecdote learned about affront to basic human dignity, to privacy and to confidentiality. It made her realize how many times on ward rounds – clerking patients or breaking bad news, especially to deaf elderly patients – doctors must throw away any regard for confidentiality without even noticing it.

Whilst a long-held ethical touchstone, confidentiality is also threatened by modern medical practices, such as the increasing emphasis on teamwork (since the doctor must of necessity share information with other health professionals), appropriate accountability to managers, and the use of computers.

Maintaining good medical practice

Doctors are expected to maintain their competence through continuing professional development and lifelong learning. The profession must be able to guarantee the competence of its members through, for example, clinical audit, peer review and revalidation. But continuing professional development is an issue that is much broader than continuing education, and involves personal growth as attention to and satisfaction with professional work. The doctor must cultivate a concern for clinical standards, and the efficiency and effectiveness of his or her actions, and pay attention to the outcomes of care.

With the ever growing range of demands on doctors linked to technological advances and increasing complexity in medicine and health care, it is increasingly difficult for the individual doctor to meet them all. The ability to

---

Box 3.13   Confidentiality

A doctor describes being taught about privacy while sharing a gynaecology ward with a particular patient.

The patient stood out from other women on the ward: she was very skinny, wore improbably high platform shoes and tight jeans, and had rather disorderly make-up and hair.

"Ello', she said, as the doctor slid further down under the covers to avoid conversation. The track marks on the girl's arms caught the doctor's eye. 'I'm in 'ere with gallstones. But its OK. They ain't going to operate. They're going to wait for me to piss them out like normal. But I ain't got nowhere to go, so they're having to find me a place in an 'ostel. Been working down King's Cross, but my boyfriend threw me out. So I got another one, but 'e ain't even been to visit me yet. Bastard. What are you in 'ere for?'

Time passed with an endless stream of assorted doctors and others picking up notes and drawing the curtains around a bed for a clerking or private discussion with the patient.

Soon the doctor knew all about the girl's real problems; it was impossible to avoid overhearing bedside consultations and inter-professional discussions at the nursing station. After the worker from the drug dependency unit visited, the doctor also knew the story behind her track marks.

The girl obviously had no idea that at least five other patients could hear every word of her conversations behind the curtain whether they wanted to or not. The people talking to her also failed to realize that other patients could overhear. The curtains seemed to provide some false sense of confidentiality. The nurse's handover also rang out around the ward: an audible summary of every patient, updated daily. The doctor then realized that everyone must have heard all about her.

(Adapted from: Steele A. Curtains for confidentiality. *BMJ* 2001; **322**: 1532.)

---

work in a team, so that all the available skills (including those of professions other than medicine) are used to the full, becomes crucial. This need not and must not be at the expense of the doctor–patient relationship.

RATIONING

There is an unwritten contract between doctors and their patients to provide optimal care, but this also has to be within available resources. The use of a particular resource for one patient denies the use of that resource for another. But doctors are increasingly concerned with health, as well as illness, not only in the individual but in the community at large – the population or public health perspective. Doctors also have contracts with their employers. In any conflict priority should be given to the patient.

Many doctors find themselves torn between two contradictory principles. On the one hand they must do the best for each individual patient. On the other hand, a resource or budget used in one way for one patient is not available for use by somebody else. A particular budget may be insufficient for the best care for each individual patient. All health care systems have to grapple with the problem of how best to allocate scarce resources. Indeed, it could be said that there has always been rationing in the NHS (see Box 3.14). Yet in no

---

Box 3.14   Mechanisms of rationing

Deterrence	Making it more difficult, e.g. • Prescription charges • GP receptionist • Appointments
Delay	Waiting lists
Deflection	Persuade others to fund, e.g. • Private • Social Services Department
Dilution	Reduction of quality, e.g. • Cheaper alternative • Less effective alternative
Denial	Refusal or termination of treatment, e.g. • Doctors decide on investigation or treatment • Medical decision on discharge date

---

country is there a clear and publicly accepted set of principles that can determine who gets what health care and when.[8]

The currently stated principles of our National Health Service, reflecting the ideas at its founding in 1948, are that the NHS should be a service available to all on the basis of clinical need, regardless of the ability to pay. The NHS should provide patients with treatment and care which is clinically effective and a good use of taxpayers' money. The service should not only be responsive in meeting the needs of individual patients, but also be capable of changing as needs change and as technology advances.

Our NHS has a limited budget of over £40 billion. The Department of Health issues an annual set of priorities, usually reflecting the concerns of the government of the day. Clinicians, purchasers, general practitioners and providers are given considerable freedom and discretion, resulting in rationing of care by rules that differ, may be incoherent and are usually implicit. As a result policy tends to emerge almost as a by-product of these individual decisions, and NHS patients get unequal access to care. This also leads to inefficiency. The rationing debate is profoundly unscientific. Evidence-based rationing requires the careful measurement of costs and health outcomes. Until principles of rationing are established and measurement is improved, the allocation of NHS resources is likely to continue to be inequitable and inefficient. This point was made as long ago as 1971 by Archie Cochrane, first President of the Faculty of Public Health Medicine and the man who gave his name to the Cochrane Database of Systematic Reviews, now a centrepiece of the approach to evidence-based health care (see Box 3.15).[9]

This view is that inefficiency is unethical. One element, sometimes considered inefficient and therefore rationing by delay, is the time it takes for effective interventions to be adopted in routine clinical practice. The classical example is the prevention of scurvy in seamen (see Box 3.16). In 1601 an English sea captain carried out an experiment and demonstrated that scurvy (a disease marked by bleeding and sponginess of gums, due to lack of fresh

---

Box 3.15   Allocation of NHS resources

'If we are ever to get the "optimum" results from our national expenditure on the NHS we must finally be able to express the results in the form of the benefit and the cost to the population of a particular type of activity, and the increased benefit that would be obtained if more money were made available.'

(From Cochrane AL. *Effectiveness and Efficiency: Random Reflections on Health Services* (Rock Carling Fellowship, 1971). London: The Nuffield Provincial Hospitals Trust; 1972.[10])

Box 3.16   Scurvy: from evidence to policy

1601	Experimental evidence available	
		146 years
1747	Evidence confirmed	
		48 years
1795	British Navy policy of supplying citrus fruits on long sea voyages	
		70 years
1865	Board of Trade policy for Merchant Navy	

A total of 264 years after empirical proof was available

---

fruit and vegetables and consequently of vitamin C) could be prevented by giving sailors three teaspoons of lemon juice every day. At that time scurvy killed more sailors on long sea voyages than warfare, accidents and all other causes of death. Nearly 150 years later this finding was confirmed by a British Navy physician, but it was a further 48 years before the British Navy eradicated scurvy by adopting the idea of supplying citrus fruits. It was a further 70 years before this became British Board of Trade policy and the Merchant Navy could cease to suffer unknown numbers of deaths (usually a half or two thirds of all long voyage sailors). Thus a total of 264 years elapsed between empirical proof being available, and the widespread implementation of a preventive treatment.

An alternative argument is that rationing need not and should not be considered until the ineffective and inefficient management of clinical resources in the health service is ironed out. It is believed that there are considerable opportunities for price control in the NHS. If all this were achieved then resources would be released for redeployment elsewhere, and could be sufficient to eliminate any need to ration effective health care, at least in the short- or medium-term future.[10]

In addition, it can be argued that existing services could be provided with improved efficiency. Services that are of no proven benefit might not be offered. Academic approaches suggest better targeting of resources to achieve best value for money. For instance, the benefits of thrombolysis treatment in coronary heart disease have been well known since the 1970s. Yet a recent survey in one health region showed that less than half the patients who could benefit were receiving this treatment.

Targeting ought to be aided by considering quality of life dimensions. Despite widespread agreement on the need to consider quality of life in health care decisions, there is little agreement over which of the large list of measures should be used. There is no agreement over whose values should be incorporated in the measures, and how different values should be weighted.[11] Health is a function of both length of life and quality of life. One of these measures, the quality-adjusted life-year (QALY), has been developed in an attempt to combine the value of these attributes into a single index number. Patient welfare is considered to be the product of length of life and the quality of that life of a particular person. The QALY approach also allows the aggregation of health gains from many patients, thus allowing the comparison of the outcomes of different interventions for a particular patient.

A targeted approach should also operate to reduce variations which remain widespread. Studies frequently show variations in access to or take up of effective interventions to be at least twofold, and often much greater.

There are also two options heard not infrequently in the public political arena. Firstly, resources could be redeployed from public services considered of a lower priority; the national defence budget is usually cited as the potential source of these resources. Secondly, taxes could be raised. This would mean in effect redeploying resources from goods and services that people buy for themselves.

The Oregon experiment

Nearly 15 years ago the state of Oregon attracted worldwide interest when it began an ambitious attempt to set priorities for health care based on a systematic basis. This started as a result of a death of a 7-year-old boy who had been waiting for a bone marrow transplant operation, and it was led by a doctor turned politician. Oregon passed legislation in 1989 designed to provide access to health insurance for all residents. A key part of the strategy was to increase eligibility for Medicaid, a publicly funded programme of health care for people with low incomes. It sought to ensure that Medicaid recipients were, whenever possible, enrolled in managed care plans. What attracted most interest was the attempt to define the basic health care package by restricting the services that would be funded. The task of determining what should be on the list was put in the hands of a health commission of 11 members comprising both professional and lay people. The work of the commission was conducted in public, and included considering the advice of experts and consulting with the community.

The Oregon health plan achieved success in some areas but failed in others. By including more people in the Medicaid health plan, the proportion of the population who were uninsured (and therefore without health care cover) was reduced from 18% in 1993 to 11% in 1996.[12] One of the most important lessons learned is considered to be that explicit priority setting tends to result in inflation of a basic health care package.

Some of the problems associated with rationing

The debate over rationing should not be confused with the debates over effectiveness and efficiency. Few people disagree with the need to increase

---

Box 3.17   Health gain criteria

Appropriateness:
To what extent is a significant health need addressed?

Quantity:
How many people will benefit?

Quality:
Effect on the quality of life (physical, mental, social, self-care, perception of pain, sense of well-being)?

Effectiveness:
Evidence of effectiveness?

Empowerment:
To what extent will the control of local people be strengthened?

Access:
Will it be inaccessible?

Acceptability:
Will it improve things?

Efficiency:
To what extent is the proposed service an efficient means for delivering these gains?

Opportunity costs:
What will not get done as a result?

---

effectiveness, and there is little controversy about denying ineffective treatments.[13] However, despite the attractiveness of and clamour sometimes for explicit approaches to rationing, there are some implications and dangers.

Experience with explicit approaches, such as the Oregon plan described above, or other approaches to public involvement such as citizen juries, may mean that the time taken for public involvement could lead to an approach being unresponsive, both to rapid changes in medical knowledge, and variations in patients' preferences and tastes. Some people care less about treatment than others; these people may be excluded from benefit, and hence the risk of social conflict. Such social judgements may also be subject to and confused with subjective judgements of medical necessity. There is therefore a need in such explicit approaches to guard against unconscious preferences that may reflect class, sex, or other social biases.

Another serious risk from explicit approaches to rationing is the potential for violating the trust between doctor and patient. It is this trust that holds the present system intact, so anything that threatens this should be avoided.

Any approach to rationing, e.g. when considering the introduction of a new service, ought to be tested against health gain criteria (see Box 3.17).

THE RESPONSIBILITY FOR TEACHING AND TRAINING

As if these fundamental and heavy duties and responsibilities are not enough, all doctors have two other imperatives they must fulfil. They have a responsibility to contribute to the training of the next generation of doctors. They also have a duty to add to the knowledge base of the discipline.

A LIFE OUTSIDE MEDICINE

In the past there has been a prevailing view that those entering the profession should commit their working lives to the service of patients. Medicine was viewed as a job which should not be constrained by strict working hours or subject to demarcation disputes. There was an inevitable impact on family life, friends and social activities. The shifting views of society now mean that young doctors want a life outside of medicine. This challenge to the conventional view of professionalism is not new. In the mid-1960s and -1970s the tone changed, and professionalism as a concept was viewed as being flawed, not least because of the conflict between altruism and self-interest.[14]

PRIVATE MEDICAL PRACTICE

More recently this debate has resurfaced over the question of private medical practice. The right to undertake private medical practice has existed for doctors since the inception of the NHS.

General practitioners are currently independent practitioners who contract singly or in groups to health authorities to provide general medical services for patients, usually in a defined area. Provided that they meet these contractual responsibilities they are free to undertake private practice as well. In reality, apart from in London, there are few general practitioners with any significant number of private patients. The independent practitioner status is being increasingly questioned because of the growing requirements of the NHS structures, processes and regulations, and because there is an increasing reluctance among new general practitioners to take on the full range of these responsibilities, which may include a very large financial investment in the premises owned by a practice.

For hospital consultants, the issues involved in private practice are much more emotive. Consultants are able to hold one of three contracts as employees of the NHS; few consultants practice totally in the private sector (see Box 3.18). A new contract is being considered.

A potential for conflict in these arrangements is perceived by many inside and outside the service. For example, waiting lists have bedevilled the NHS

Box 3.18   NHS consultants and private practice

1. Consultants with a full-time NHS contract will normally not undertake any private practice
2. Consultants with a maximum part-time contract may normally undertake private practice in their own time up to a maximum of 10% of their NHS income
3. Consultants may work part-time in a proportion agreed with their employer and be free to work in the private sector in the rest of their time

since its inception; waiting lists virtually do not exist in any other health system. Waiting lists and waiting times have increasingly become a focus for the governments of the day and of whatever political persuasion. The conflict of interest perceived in NHS consultants being allowed to take on private practice is the possibility that there is a perverse incentive for them. The idea is that there is a value to a consultant in having a long waiting list for patients either to be seen or to have a particular operation, since this is more likely to push a patient into wanting to see the consultant, or have the operation, privately, to the obvious financial advantage of the consultant.

A CULTURE FOR THE NHS OF THE FUTURE

In July 2001 the Bristol Royal Infirmary Inquiry report was published.[15] The Inquiry looked at events at the Bristol Royal Infirmary between 1984 and 1995 where between 30 and 35 more children, aged under 1 year, died after open heart surgery than was typical of similar units elsewhere in England. The events at Bristol and the recommendations made in the report have already been a major catalyst for change in the NHS. The view at the time was that the ingredients that led to the excess deaths in Bristol were present throughout the NHS. The report paints a clear picture of what is needed (see Box 3.19). Nearly 200 recommendations were made, and some have already been implemented.

Box 3.19   The Bristol Royal Infirmary Inquiry Report[16]

The culture required in the NHS:

- A culture of safety
- A culture of quality
- Openness
- Accountability
- A culture of public service
- A culture in which collaborative teamwork is prized
- A culture of flexibility in which innovation can flourish in response to patients' needs
- Outcomes can be monitored and evaluated
- Staff are well regulated, trained and supported
- Error is minimized, but where it does occur lessons are learnt and shared
- Patients are genuine partners in the decision-making process.

Patients should be entitled to expect:

- Respect and honesty
- Care in a setting which is well led
- Competent health care professionals
- Care which is safe
- Care of an appropriate standard
- Inclusion and involvement in the NHS, both as patients and as members of the public.

Box 3.20   Human values

Creativity
The habit of truth
The sense of human dignity
Tenderness
Kindliness
Human intimacy and love

(After: Bronowski J. *Science and Human Values*. Middlesex: Pelican Books, 1964.)

CONCLUSION

It is not possible to consider medicine's core values without setting them in the context of human values (Box 3.20). Bronowski described three: creativity, the habit of truth, and the sense of human dignity; to which he added the human value of tenderness, of kindliness, of human intimacy and love.[16] Professionalism in medicine is an ideal to be pursued because it can lead to ever higher standards which, by being constantly aimed at, lead to higher levels of performance.[17] This is at the heart of clinical governance.

REFERENCES

1. Spence J. *The Purpose and Practice of Medicine*. Oxford: Oxford University Press, 1960.
2. Smith R. Medicine's core values. *BMJ* 1994; **309**: 1247–1248.
3. Irvine DH. The performance of doctors. I: Professionalism and self regulation in a changing world. *BMJ* 1997; **314**: 1540–1542.
4. Parsons T. *The Social System*. Illinois: The Free Press, 1951.
5. Calman K. The profession of medicine. *BMJ* 1994; **309**; 1140–1143.
6. Szasz TS, Hollander M. *Arch Intern Med* 1956; **97**: 585.
7. Core Values Conference. *Core Values for the Medical Profession in the 21st Century*. London: BMA, 1995.
8. Maynard A. Rationing health care. *BMJ* 1996; **313**: 1499.
9. Cochrane AL. *Effectiveness and Efficiency: Random Reflections on Health Services* (Rock Carling Fellowship, 1971). London: Nuffield Provincial Hospitals Trust, 1972.
10. Roberts CJ, Crosby DL. Anti-Rationing Group also wants to contribute to the debate. *BMJ* 1996; **313**: 557.
11. Cairns J. Measuring health outcomes. *BMJ* 1996; **313**: 6.
12. Ham C. Retracing the Oregon trail: the experience of rationing and the Oregon health plan. *BMJ* 1998; **316**: 1956–1959.
13. Smith R. Rationing health care: moving the debate forward. *BMJ* 1996; **312**: 1553–1554.
14. Friedson E. *Profession of Medicine: A Study of the Sociology of Applied Knowledge*. New York: Dodd and Mead,1970.
15. Public Inquiry into Children's Heart Surgery at the Bristol Royal Infirmary 1984–1995. *Learning from Bristol*. London: Stationery Office, 2001 (Cmnd 5207).
16. Bronowski J. *Science and Human Values*. Middlesex: Pelican Books, 1964.
17. Cruess SR, Cruess RL. Professionalism must be taught. *BMJ* 1997; **315**: 1674–1677.

Clinical effectiveness and evidence-based practice

4

'One of the chief causes of poverty in science is imaginary wealth. The aim of science is not to open the door to infinite wisdom, but to set a limit to infinite error.'

Bertolt Brecht

This chapter describes the development of lifelong learning and evidence-based practice. The following areas are covered:

- Lifelong learning
- Clinical effectiveness
- Randomized controlled trials and systematic reviews
- Evidence-based practice
- Searching the evidence
- Appraising the evidence
- Presenting the evidence.

LIFELONG LEARNING

Health care used to be simple, largely ineffective and mostly safe. Over the last 50 years it has become complex, more effective, but also more dangerous. *Lifelong learning* (learning how to learn all through our life) describes the continuous process of keeping up-to-date with the rapidly changing nature of health care. It promotes skills regarding how to learn rather than what to learn, so that we can cope with the complexity of the changing knowledge base and ensure safe and effective clinical practice. Lifelong learning has developed to cope with the rapidly growing volume of knowledge and the recognition that our traditional methods of learning need to adapt.

1. *Too much to learn, too easy to forget.* There are over 2 million biomedical research papers published each year in over 25 000 journals. The number of published papers is doubling every 16 years, so a newly qualified health professional will be faced with the unenviable task of trying to make sense of over 8 million research papers per year by the time she retires. This creates two problems: the volume of medical information to contend with and its rapidly changing nature.

Clearly the days of the omniscient doctor leaving medical school with his 'bible' to see him through his professional career are long gone (if they ever existed). As well as facing rapidly changing treatments and practice, our minds are not designed as CD-ROMs to store huge databases of 'answers'. We are human and we forget. This can have its advantages (grievances, out-of-date medical practice) but for most health professionals this outcome is potentially dangerous. One study in North America found that whether or not you had your hypertension treated correlated more with your doctor's year of graduation than the degree of end-organ damage.

2. *Ineffective learning methods.* Just by reading this sentence you show you are the wrong reader. It is likely that this book will preach to the converted rather than deal with getting information to those professionals who most need it. Like most continuing professional and medical education, there is a strong element of self-selection. We can determine from research studies that continuing professional education works if you do not want it, and if you do want it you don't need it. Similarly, it is likely that the books we read reflect our own particular interests rather than our educational needs. This becomes almost an inverse need law with professional development – we learn more and more about less and less.

The other mainstay of traditional professional development, the lecture, is also of dubious value in developing up-to-date clinicians. Again there is self-selection in those who attend. Its didactic format then assumes that health professionals are empty vessels just waiting to be filled with the endless words of knowledge from the relevant expert in a dark, sleep-inducing lecture theatre.

The foundation for lifelong learning is having the confidence to recognize our educational needs. This is more of an attitude than a skill. We must recognize that much of what we think is correct may not be so and we should be prepared to be more open to explore better practice. Like the recovering alcoholic in admitting a problem, we need to be proud of standing up and saying 'I don't know'. The alternative, to pretend, to cover up, to bluff, is no longer an acceptable option.

As well as encouraging greater recognition of our own learning needs and how to deal with them, we must also ensure that the environments in which we work are supportive and conducive to learning. This is not just the responsibility of the doctor or nurse. We must move away from the notion of finger-pointing and blame, to one of shared responsibility for the professional, the patient and the organization.

The next stage is to know where to look for the answer to the particular clinical problem and then how to decide whether or not that answer is valid and appropriate to your patient. The rest of this chapter will concentrate on the basis of the knowledge that informs our clinical decisions (the evidence) and the skills needed to find and appraise this evidence in order to support lifelong learning (critical appraisal).

EVIDENCE OF EFFECTIVENESS: DOES IT WORK?

One of the key principles of a good quality health service is that medical and health care interventions should be effective. Effectiveness describes the extent to which treatments (such as drugs, operations or counselling) improve health outcomes of patients in clinical practice. Most patients, and indeed doctors, assume that everything we do in clinical practice is effective – why else would we be doing it? However, it has been estimated that up to 80% of medical interventions are of uncertain benefit and continue as rituals of practice more through history than science.

In order to find out if a treatment is effective we need to evaluate its benefit (or harm) in a clinical trial. This can be a trial on a single patient; for example, giving a patient with multiple sclerosis a course of steroids and following them up a month later to find out if they feel better or have had improvement in their disability. This anecdotal observation is often the basis of decision-making in our clinical practice careers. If the patient returns the next month and reports that they feel greatly improved, it may be tempting to pat your-self on the back and bask in reflected glory; however, there are a number of explanations that may account for her improvement.

1. Temporal changes. The disease is a relapsing and remitting disease and this episode may have got better without any treatment. Similarly self-limiting diseases such as sore throats will resolve with or without antibiotics.
2. Placebo effect. Every drug can exert a placebo effect, and every doctor can exert a halo effect to improve the reported health of patients. Not only can placebos lead to improvements in health outcomes, but patients will report side effects from these inactive preparations. Drug companies are never shy about advertising that 30% of patients got better on their new Fabulosa drug, but rarely admit that 20% got better on the chalk tablets in the control group.
3. Reporting bias. Patients will often report improvement to the doctor because that is what they think the doctor wants to hear, and they do not want to disappoint. The doctor on the other hand can exert an observation bias by recording clinical improvement in line with their prior prejudice.

RANDOMIZED CONTROLLED TRIALS

Historically, clinical practice relied heavily on anecdotal evaluations like Rush's (Box 4.1). However, the science of clinical trials improved with the rational observations of doctors such as Louis and by 1948 the first ran-domized clinical trial was copied from methods used by agriculturalists to evaluate crop rotations and conducted to demonstrate the effectiveness of streptomycin in the treatment of tuberculosis.

Clinical effectiveness and evidence-based practice

Box 4.1   Clinical trials before 1950

- Rush (1790) – Notes in his diary reporting the effectiveness of bloodletting for yellow fever:

- '... never before did I experience such sublime joy as when I saw the effectiveness of drawing the blood. The reader will wonder when I add an extract from my notebook dated 10th September: "Thank God. Of the 100 patients whom I visited this day, I have lost none".'

- Pierre-Charles-Alexandre Louis. A Parisian doctor who undertook one of the first controlled trials to evaluate the effectiveness of bloodletting for the treatment of pneumonia. He found that 18/29 (62%) of patients who were bled died, compared with 9/27 (33%) of the control patients who were not bled. Although he had no X-rays to confirm his diagnosis, and there was no randomization, this provided evidence about the lack of clinical value of bloodletting.

Using a control group with a comparable placebo can allow for temporal and placebo effects to be measured and compared to the treatment under evaluation. By randomizing patients to either the treatment under evaluation or the control arm, the potential for selection bias is removed and patients in both groups should end up with similar characteristics. Non-randomized trials may overestimate the size of effect of treatments by 40%. By blinding the trialists and the patients to which arm they were in, observation bias can be reduced. Trials that are not blinded may overestimate the size of effect by 20%.

Some interventions are so dramatically or obviously effective that observation can be sufficient to confirm benefit. For example, when penicillin was first evaluated in North Africa in World War II, medics gave it to the most severely ill patients and the healthier patients acted as controls. It was so effective that despite this selection bias in favour of the control group, the penicillin group had a lower mortality rate. Other interventions such as general anaesthesia or cardiopulmonary resuscitation are so dramatic in their effect that more rigorous trials are not necessary (or ethically feasible).

Many people would consider the randomized controlled trial to be one of the greatest contributions to health care over the last 50 years. It provides us with the best trial evidence and has allowed us to confirm the effectiveness of many existing and new treatments, and confirmed the uselessness of others (see Box 4.2).

Box 4.2   Randomized controlled trials

Importance of a placebo control
Gastric freezing became a popular treatment for duodenal ulcer in the 1960s after it was shown to relieve pain in a case series of 31 patients. A subsequent placebo-controlled trial showed that the same proportion of patients in the placebo group obtained relief of their pain due to the psychological effect of the procedure.

Importance of choosing the right outcome
In the 1980s patients with frequent ventricular ectopics after a heart attack were found to have a high risk of death and a randomized controlled trial showed that the anti-arrhythmic drugs flecainide and enconide reduced the frequency of these ectopics. After

---

these had been put into widespread clinical practice, a subsequent randomized controlled trial showed that patients who received these drugs actually had a greater risk of dying than those who did not. Clinical and patient-based outcomes should be used rather than physiological outcomes.

Importance of observation bias
Laparoscopic cholecystectomy has been shown in a number of randomized controlled trials to lead to shorter stays in hospital and a quicker return to work. In the 1990s a trial attempted to introduce blinding by separating the surgeon in the theatre from the surgeon making the decision on the wards. All the patients were given large, blood-stained bandages to prevent the surgeon on the ward identifying who had had keyhole surgery. No difference was found in postoperative duration of stay or speed of return to work.

SYSTEMATIC REVIEWS

Since the first such trial in 1948 there have been almost a million randomized controlled trials evaluating thousands of different medical interventions. Settings range from Bradford to Borneo with many variations of the patients included and the exact type of treatment given. Many of these trials have been small and have not had the statistical power to provide a definitive treatment effect. Many lie unpublished or lost in obscure journals. Some will show benefit from a particular treatment, whereas others may show harm.

If we are to find out whether or not a treatment is effective then we need to summarize the evidence from these different trials. Traditional reviews of the published evidence have usually relied on experts or researchers in the field to tell us the answer. However, this method has two main weaknesses:

1. The reviewer may have a particular prejudice or prior belief. They may want to push their own contribution to the research evidence as the answer, or may want to put down rivals. They may want to canvass for funding for a particular research project that comes out of their conclusions.
2. The review may miss trials that can contribute to the answer. Simply searching Medline will miss a third of randomized controlled trials. Many trials will be published in the form of conference abstracts or research theses and never make it into journal print – this is called the grey literature.

Then there is the *Tower of Babel* bias where non-English language researchers will tend to publish dramatic results in the prestigious English language journals, but if the trial shows no benefit it may get confined to the *Hungarian Medical Journal*, lost forever in translation. Up to 40% of stroke intervention trials are in Japanese journals and can quite easily be ignored if no effort is made to translate them.

Many trials end up not being published at all. *Publication bias* describes how journal editors favour trials that show positive results, and tend to be left cold by trials that show no effect. So the published literature tends to show positive results and ignores neutral or negative results. Lastly, many

Clinical effectiveness and evidence-based practice

trials never get to the stage of even being submitted, either because the researcher moves on to other jobs or just through lack of time. Again, this *bottom drawer bias* tends to happen more often if the trial shows no result, or negative results.

So many traditional reviews end up being haphazard and biased, and it has been shown that the majority have inappropriate or misleading conclusions. Systematic reviews have developed from the recognition that summaries of the evidence need to be objective and unbiased. A number of steps are taken to ensure that the review is systematic:

- Clear and precise objectives stated for the review so that the review addresses a clear question.
- An explicit and rigorous search of the published and grey literature including writing to relevant experts in the field to find unpublished evidence.
- Explicit inclusion and exclusion criteria for trials to be included in the review.
- Transparent appraisal of trials and consistent data extraction.
- Clear methods of combining results, either through statistical techniques such as meta-analysis, or a more narrative description of the evidence.

The results of these reviews can then be used to provide a valid basis for informing clinical practice and identifying gaps in the research that should be addressed in future trials (Box 4.3).

An international network of clinicians and researchers was established in the 1990s to provide up-to-date and accessible summaries of all randomized controlled trials of medical and health care interventions. The *Cochrane Collaboration* is named after Archie Cochrane, an early advocate for clinical effectiveness in health services. The Collaboration publishes systematic reviews on all clinical areas on the Cochrane Library, a quarterly CD-ROM that aims to provide the best single source of reliable evidence about the effects of health care. This is discussed later in this chapter.

Box 4.3   Examples of systematic reviews that have challenged conventional practice

1. Nebulizers have long been used for the treatment of acute asthma in the belief that they were more effective than simple, hand-held inhalers. A systematic review of the 16 trials comparing the two drug delivery devices showed that simple inhalers were just as effective as nebulizers in treating acute exacerbations of asthma.

2. Human albumin solution is widely used for the emergency treatment of shock to restore blood volume. A systematic review and meta-analysis of 30 trials evaluating the effectiveness of albumin found that not only was there no evidence of its effectiveness but there was a strong suggestion that its use might increase the risk of death.

3. Psychological counselling and debriefing after traumatic events has become common practice. However, a systematic review of the eight randomized trials evaluating the effectiveness of psychological debriefing found no evidence that it was useful as a treatment for prevention of subsequent post-traumatic stress disorder.

EVIDENCE-BASED PRACTICE

We can now classify different research into a hierarchy of evidence (Table 4.1). This attempts to describe the validity and reliability of research evidence from the anecdotal through to the 'gold standard' randomized controlled trial and beyond to a systematic review of all relevant randomized controlled trials.

This type of hierarchy is now commonly used to describe the level of evidence in support of guidelines, recommendations and review conclusions. These levels are described as in a 1–5 or ABC classification and help to clarify which clinical recommendations are based on expert opinion and which are based on the best scientific research evidence. This not only increases the transparency of clinical decision-making, but can also help clinicians and their patients to make informed choices about health care.

Linking the principles behind lifelong learning to an explicit categorization of the strength of research evidence has provided the basis for *evidence-based medicine or practice*. David Sackett, one of the leading proponents of evidence-based practice has defined this as 'a process of life-long, self-directed learning which integrates the best up-to-date evidence with individual expertise'.

Evidence-based practice aims to incorporate the systematic, explicit and judicious use of best research evidence into routine patient care. There are few treatments that are 100% safe and 100% effective. Most fall into a much greyer area where some patients will benefit and some will have side effects. Evidence-based practice attempts to acknowledge some of this uncertainty.

There are five key steps for evidence-based practice (Figure 4.1):

- Form an answerable question. This requires clinical decisions to be broken down into specific components that can then be addressed. So rather than 'Should I anticoagulate this patient in atrial fibrillation?' the question should be 'Will the benefits of warfarin in reducing the risk of stroke outweigh the harms from bleeding in this 85-year-old woman with hypertension?' The latter defines the patient, the treatment, the desired outcome and the potential harm.
- Track down the best evidence. This is discussed in the next section. For the question asked above we can find a systematic review of all the randomized controlled trials demonstrating that elderly people with

Table 4.1 Classification of evidence according to its quality, reliability and validity

Evidence	Classification
1 A systematic review of at least two randomized controlled trials	BEST
2 A randomized, controlled trial	
3 A cohort study	
4 A case-control study	
5 An uncontrolled study with dramatic results	
6 An expert committee report or similar	
7 Anecdotal evidence	WORST

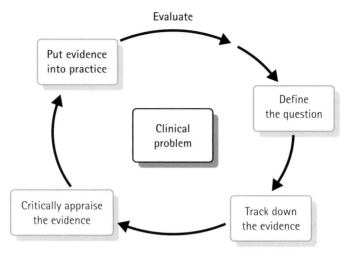

Evaluate

Put evidence
into practice

Define
the question

Clinical
problem

Critically appraise
the evidence

Track down
the evidence

Fig. 4.1   Cycle for evidence-based practice.

atrial fibrillation and a risk factor for stroke have a 68% reduced risk of
stroke on warfarin relative to placebo (4.4% absolute risk reduction).
- Critically appraise the evidence. What are the results? Are the results of
  the systematic review valid? Are they applicable to my 85-year-old
  patient? This is discussed below.
- Apply the evidence. Put your evidence-based decision into practice in
  consultation with your patient. Let her know about the potential benefits
  of warfarin and the potential harms of side effects. In the past this was
  always a decision for the clinician – 'doctor knows best'. As patients
  become more empowered and knowledgeable, the decision should
  become their own. User-friendly methods for presenting results to help
  patients understand the risks and benefits of treatment are becoming
  more available (Box 4.4).

Box 4.4   Added advantages in practising evidence-based medicine

For individuals
- Enables clinicians to upgrade their knowledge base routinely
- Improves clinicians' understanding of research methods and makes them more critical in
  using data
- Improves confidence in management decisions
- Improves computer literacy and data searching techniques
- Improves reading habits

For clinical teams
- Gives team a framework for group problem solving and for teaching
- Enables juniors to contribute usefully to team

For patients
- More effective use of resources
- Better communication with patients about the rationale behind management decisions

- Evaluate performance. Auditing our own practice against the evidence is important to show how we perform over time. It allows us to demonstrate good quality care and identify problems and gaps in performance over time. Clinical audit will be discussed in Chapter 6.

Evidence-based practice integrates lifelong learning with up-to-date knowledge. It can also improve our understanding of research and clinical trials. Rather than just relying on second-hand interpretations of the evidence, or bottom-line conclusions from the abstracts of clinical papers, it encourages us to be more questioning about research methodologies and results. It promotes confidence in clinical decision-making when we do reach an answer that we know is based on the best science available rather than a distant memory.

The main disadvantage of evidence-based practice is that it is potentially very time-consuming. Try undergoing the five steps for every clinical decision you make during a day and you may find yourself looking up Medline all night. There are a number of more realistic ways of incorporating evidence-based practice into routine clinical practice. Searching and appraising the research evidence can be limited to key clinical problems, once a week for instance, to promote a method of self-directed learning. It can form the basis of journal clubs – allowing real clinical questions to drive the agenda rather than random papers. Alternatively you can rely on others to search and appraise the evidence to provide answers, for example, by using the Cochrane Library or Clinical Evidence.

There is also a tension between qualitative and quantitative research. Randomized controlled trials may indeed provide the best, objective evidence of treatments in diabetes. However, care needs to be taken not to over-rely on methods that may include only a narrow patient group, and tend to be dominated by pharmaceutical interventions. Other research methods such as qualitative research and observational studies can provide a valuable balance between internal validity of evidence from a trial and the external validity to everyday clinical practice. It is important to ensure that similar standards of critical appraisal are still applied.

The other main problem with evidence-based practice is the lack of evidence. Frequently the trials necessary to answer a clinical question have not been done, or if they have, they have measured biomedical outcomes rather than patient outcomes. Too much previous research has been haphazard and disconnected from clinical reality. Researchers have often been driven more through pet interests than health service priorities. By defining gaps in the research evidence after searching and appraising the literature, we can identify what research studies need to be carried out and encourage funding bodies to commission these.

SEARCHING FOR EVIDENCE

With so many research studies published and so many more to come, trying to find the right evidence is a new skill that all health professionals need to master. Without a clear understanding of where to look and how to search, it is easy to drown in the ocean of mediocre literature. Most hospitals and districts have a team of expert medical or health librarians and every clinician should seek out their help and support in tracking down the right evidence. Rigorous searching can require complex step-wise interrogation of numerous databases using a panoply of search terms. This is best left to the experts. But all of us need to master the basic skills.

There are various databases to search and which one you choose will depend on how much time you have and how in-depth you want to go.

1. The main library databases include *Medline*, which is North American; *Embase*, which is European; and *CINAHL*, which has a nursing/therapy emphasis. Medline is the most popular medical database. It contains millions of references categorized by time (e.g. 1987–1992), clinical area and study design. Relevant studies can be searched by combining the clinical topic (using text words or MESH headings) and the appropriate trial design to find the best evidence. Different questions require different trial designs. For example:

   • Studies of treatments should be limited to randomized controlled trials
   • Studies of diagnostic tests should be limited to cross-sectional studies
   • Studies of prognosis should be limited to inception cohorts.

   If no studies are found then the search can be broadened. If too many are found then they can be limited by making the search terms more specific.

   The problem with using databases such as Medline is that you may miss many relevant trials that are mis-classified (for example, about a third of randomized controlled trials will be missed), or be swamped by irrelevant papers. To be confident about your search terms and search strategy you also need to be well-trained and a regular user. So alternative places to search may be better.

2. A number of journals are now acting as filters to try and pick out all the high quality, rigorous clinical research evidence from the mountains of curriculum vitae-enhancing rubbish. Journals such as *ACP Journal Club* and *Evidence Based Medicine* screen all the major clinical journals for studies that fulfil clear criteria for validity and reliability of methods and results. Less than 1% of papers meet these criteria, but this research 'cream' can provide an excellent source of evidence about therapies, diagnostic tests, prognosis, causation, quality improvement, professional development, economic appraisals and systematic reviews.

   These summaries have been collated since 1991 to form *Best Evidence*. This is available on CD-ROM and in health libraries.

   Another international collaboration is *Clinical Evidence*. This is produced by the BMJ Publishing Group and the American College of Physicians. It aims to provide an up-to-date (published every 6 months) compendium of the best available evidence on the effects of common clinical interventions.

3. The most comprehensive source of good evidence is the Cochrane Library. The Cochrane Collaboration publishes its Database of Systematic

Reviews on all clinical areas on the Cochrane Library, a quarterly CD-ROM that aims to provide the best single source of reliable evidence about the effects of health care. Also on the library is the York Database of Reviews of Effectiveness (DARE) and a register of controlled clinical trials (to try and prevent future publication bias). Further details can be found at *www.cochrane.co.uk*.

The reviews on the Cochrane Library attempt to define the important clinical questions, undertake thorough searches for all available trials and systematically review these trials to end up with clear answers for clinicians. They are published with synopses, abstracts and full reviews, so that busy clinicians can obtain quick answers when they need them, or more in-depth discussions when appropriate. Although the Library has many gaps (either lack of reviews or lack of primary research trials), and excludes all non-randomized controlled research, it is becoming more and more useful with time, not necessarily as a clinical reference document, but as a definitive source of medical knowledge.

A prerequisite for promoting evidence-based practice is the easy accessibility of these databases. The days when medical knowledge sat in dusty bookcases in a library far removed from the wards and the clinics are over. With information networks, intranets and electronic publishing, evidence for clinical decision-making should be available wherever patients are located. Networked computers on the wards and in out-patient clinics should provide quick access to the databases above so that information is available at the right time and in the right place to support day-to-day decision-making. This aspect is discussed further in Chapter 8.

APPRAISING THE EVIDENCE

After searching for the evidence, the next step is to read it and decide on the strength and the quality of the research findings. This is often called critical appraisal. We tend to be over-simplistic in reporting research findings, categorizing them into black or white (the drug worked or it didn't). However, research results are rarely so neat and tidy. There are many grey areas around how much the treatment worked and with what harm or side effects. We must weigh up the costs and benefits to make our own decision about whether or not the treatment is suitable for our particular patient (and increasingly individual patients will want to do so themselves).

There is nothing clever about appraising a paper, although many people are unused to doing it and lack the confidence to believe their own conclusions. Just as taking a clinical history or performing a clinical examination seems complex and difficult to the novice, so can critical appraisal of a paper. The key, as with history taking or clinical examination, is to start with a clear structure. In reading a paper there are three key questions to ask:

- *Are the results valid?*
- *What are the results?*
- *Are the results applicable to my patient?*

If the study is of poor quality, with potential biases, then there is no point knowing what the results are, as they will not be valid. If the results are valid then you need to decide how appropriate they are based on the patient's values and preferences.

The more detailed questions to ask about a paper depend on what the paper is about. If it is an evaluation of a therapy then you need a randomized controlled trial with double-blinding of patients and researchers, on an appropriate population of consecutive patients in order to provide the base evidence. The following questions should be addressed (Box 4.5):

Box 4.5   Critical appraisal questions for a treatment study

	Yes	Can't tell	No
Are the results valid?			
1) Was the assignment of patients to treatments randomized?	☐	☐	☐
2) Were all patients who entered the trial properly accounted for and attributed at its conclusion?	☐	☐	☐
3) Was follow-up complete?	☐	☐	☐
4) Were patients analysed in the groups to which they were randomized?	☐	☐	☐
5) Were patients, health workers, and study personnel blinded to treatment?	☐	☐	☐
6) Were the groups similar at the start of the trial?	☐	☐	☐
7) Aside from the experimental intervention, were the groups treated equally?	☐	☐	☐
What are the results?			
1) How large was the treatment effect? (What outcomes are measured?)			
2) How precise was the treatment effect? (What are the confidence intervals?)			
Will the results help me care for my patients?			
1) Can the results be applied to my patient care?	☐	☐	☐
2) Were all clinically important outcomes considered?	☐	☐	☐
3) Are the likely benefits worth the potential harms and costs?	☐	☐	☐
4) Are patients' values and preferences addressed?	☐	☐	☐

If you want to find out about the accuracy and usefulness of a diagnostic test, or of clinical signs or symptoms, then ideally you need an independent, masked comparison with a reference standard among an appropriate population of consecutive patients. The questions that you should ask about the paper are shown in Box 4.6:

Box 4.6 Critical appraisal questions for a paper on diagnosis

	Yes	Can't tell	No

Are the results of the study valid?

1) Was there an independent, blind comparison with a reference standard? ☐ ☐ ☐

2) Did the patient sample include an appropriate spectrum of patients to whom the diagnostic test will be applied in clinical practice? ☐ ☐ ☐

3) Did the results of the test being evaluated influence the decision to perform the reference standard? ☐ ☐ ☐

4) Were the methods for performing the test described in sufficient detail to permit replication? ☐ ☐ ☐

What are the results?

1) Are likelihood ratios for the test results presented or data necessary for their calculation provided? ☐ ☐ ☐

Will the results help me in caring for my patients?

1) Will the reproducibility of the test result and its interpretation be satisfactory in my setting? ☐ ☐ ☐

2) Are the results applicable to my patient? ☐ ☐ ☐

3) Will the results change my management? ☐ ☐ ☐

4) Will patients be better off as a result of the test? ☐ ☐ ☐

Are the results of this diagnostic study valid?

1) Was there an independent, blind comparison with a reference ('gold') standard of diagnosis? ☐ ☐ ☐

2) Was the diagnostic test evaluated in an appropriate spectrum of patients (like those in whom it would be used in practice)? ☐ ☐ ☐

3) Was the reference standard applied regardless of the diagnostic test result? ☐ ☐ ☐

If you want to find out about the prognosis of a patient with a particular disease then you need a paper that reports outcomes (mortality, relapse rate) in a representative cohort of patients that have been followed up over time. The questions that should be asked are shown in Box 4.7:

Box 4.7 Critical appraisal questions for a prognosis study

	Yes	Can't tell	No

Are the results of the study valid?

Primary guides:

Was there a representative and well-defined sample of patients at a similar point in the course of the disease? ☐ ☐ ☐

Was follow-up sufficiently long and complete? ☐ ☐ ☐

Secondary guides:

Were objective and unbiased outcome
criteria used? ☐ ☐ ☐

Was there adjustment for important
prognostic factors? ☐ ☐ ☐

What are the results?

How large is the likelihood of the outcome event(s)
in a specified period of time? ☐ ☐ ☐

How precise are the estimates of likelihood? ☐ ☐ ☐

Will the results help me in caring for my patients?
Were the study patients similar to my own? ☐ ☐ ☐

Will the results lead directly to selecting or
avoiding therapy? ☐ ☐ ☐
Are the results useful for reassuring or
counselling patients? ☐ ☐ ☐

When we read a systematic review we hope that the authors have searched the literature adequately and critically appraised the studies. However, we need to be able to recognize poor quality reviews. The questions to ask about review are shown in Box 4.8:

Box 4.8   Critical appraisal questions for a review

	Yes	Can't tell	No
Are the results of the study valid?			
1 Did the review address a focused clinical question?	☐	☐	☐
2 Were the criteria used to select articles for inclusion appropriate?	☐	☐	☐
3 Is it unlikely that important, relevant studies were missed?	☐	☐	☐
4 Was the validity of the included studies appraised?	☐	☐	☐
5 Were assessments of studies reproducible?	☐	☐	☐
6 Were the results similar from study to study?	☐	☐	☐
What are the results?			
1 What are the overall results of the review?	☐	☐	☐
2 How precise were the results?	☐	☐	☐
Will the results help me in caring for my patients?			
1 Can the results be applied to my patient care?	☐	☐	☐
2 Were all clinically important outcomes considered?	☐	☐	☐
3 Are the benefits worth the harms and costs?	☐	☐	☐

PRESENTING THE EVIDENCE

The last issue to mention in this chapter is that of presentation of results. Researchers and drug companies are always keen to advertise results that grab headlines. So for example if a drug reduces the risk of 1-year mortality from coronary heart disease from 4% to 2% compared with the control group, you can be sure that the full-page colour adverts will tell you about how this wonderdrug reduces mortality by 50% – the relative risk reduction. The absolute risk reduction, however, is only 2% – not so dramatic, but much more clinically useful. A further advance on absolute risk reduction is the number needed to treat (or harm) – the NNT (or NNH). This is the inverse of the absolute risk reduction and puts the results into a more practically relevant form of patient numbers (see Box 4.9).

More recent developments in presenting results have tried to use methods that can be understood by patients themselves. There is no doubt that such informed decision-making will become more of the norm than the exception as patients become more empowered as consumers and information rich. These methods frequently use graphics such as smiley faces to represent outcomes. An example is given in Figure 4.2.

Box 4.9   What is number needed to treat?

The concept of 'number needed to treat' has become popular because it combines an estimate of the relative benefit of a particular treatment with the background risk of patients. It is the inverse of the absolute risk reduction and represents how many people would need to receive a particular treatment or intervention in order that one of them should benefit from the treatment.

A practical example can be taken from the recent concerns about third-generation oral contraceptive pills and the risk of deep vein thrombosis. It is thought that third-generation pills carry a risk of DVT of about 25 per 100 000 women per year of use; in comparison, second-generation pills carry a risk of about 15 per 100 000 women years and in women who do not take the pill the risk is about 5 per 100 000 per year.

Switching users of third-generation pills to a second-generation equivalent will result in an impressive-sounding relative risk reduction of 40%, but as the risk of DVT is so low the absolute risk reduction is only 0.0001, giving an NNT of 10 000 women needing to be changed to prevent a single DVT in 1 year.

Fig. 4.2   Use of antibiotics in acute otitis media. (a) This picture represents 100 children who are all given antibiotics for ear infections. The 86 green faces are children who would have been free from pain at 2–7 days even if they had not received an antibiotic. The 9 red faces are children who are still in pain even with antibiotics. The 5 purple faces are the only children who show a benefit; they would have been in pain without the antibiotic, but are not in pain when they receive one. Since it is not possible to identify which children will benefit, all 100 need to be given the antibiotic for 5 to benefit. This represents the number needed to treat (NNT) of 20 for a single child to benefit. (b) In contrast, this picture shows that when all 100 children are given antibiotics an extra 8 will suffer diarrhoea, vomiting or a rash. This means that the number needed to cause a harmful outcome in one child (NNH) is 12.

a)

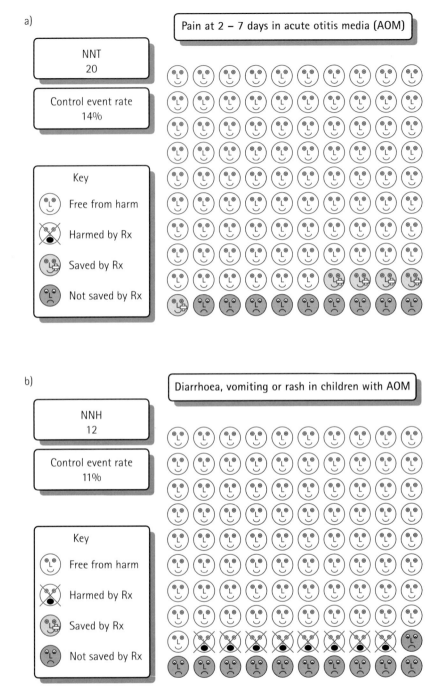

NNT
20

Control event rate
14%

Key

Free from harm

Harmed by Rx

Saved by Rx

Not saved by Rx

Pain at 2 – 7 days in acute otitis media (AOM)

b)

NNH
12

Control event rate
11%

Key

Free from harm

Harmed by Rx

Saved by Rx

Not saved by Rx

Diarrhoea, vomiting or rash in children with AOM

FURTHER READING AND INFORMATION

Cates C. http//www.mango3d.cwc.net/exam.htm

Clinical Evidence, Issue 3, BMJ Publishing Group, London June 2000.

Pencheon D, Wright J. Keeping up to date through lifelong learning. In: *The Evidence Base for Diabetes Care*. Oxford: Oxford University Press, 2002.

Sackett DL, Straus SE, Richardson WS, Rosenberg W, Haynes RB. *Evidence Based Medicine*, 2nd edn. Edinburgh: Churchill Livingstone, 2000.

Clinical effectiveness and evidence-based practice

Lifelong learning

5

'Teaching is only demonstrating that it is possible. Learning is making it possible for yourself.'

Paul Coelho: The Pilgrimage, *1987*

In this chapter we look at:

- The responsibility for keeping up to date
- Basic medical education
- General professional training
- Higher specialist training
- Lifelong learning
- The principles of learning
- The skills and competencies doctors require
- Appraisal and feedback
- Personal development planning
- Mentoring
- Continuing professional development
- Revalidation.

THE RESPONSIBILITY TO KEEP UP TO DATE

'You must keep your knowledge and skills up to date throughout your working life. In particular, you should take part regularly in educational activities which develop your competence and performance. You must work with colleagues to monitor and maintain your awareness of the quality of the care you provide. In particular, you must take part in regular and systematic medical and clinical audit, recording data honestly. Where necessary you must respond to the results of audit to improve your practice, for example by undertaking further training. You must also respond constructively to assessments and appraisals of your professional competence and performance.'[1]

Thus, all doctors have an ethical responsibility to keep up to date. This will involve maintaining and adding knowledge; maintaining, adding and refining skills; and developing professional attitudes. The effective doctor is the one who can perform to a high level of quality in areas of work that are appropriate to the post that the person holds. Different attributes and skills may be relevant in different posts and at different stages of the person's career. Learning is something one does for oneself.[2]

BASIC MEDICAL EDUCATION

Medical training in the UK is still largely based on the apprenticeship model. This begins with limited and controlled exposure and involvement. Over time there is a spectrum of increasing depth and breadth. Theoretical knowledge is gradually placed more in the context of its application to the care of patients. There is movement towards greater independence.

It is not that many years ago since it was possible to pursue any career pathway in medicine with only the basic medical degree. It was only in the mid-1970s that the Merrison report defined the concept of the 'basic educable doctor'.[3] This idea first indicated that a medical degree was merely the start of training for a career in some branch of medicine. Although many doctors recognized that they needed more training and experience and sought this out, it was not obligatory.

The purpose of basic education now is to prepare the ground for a career involving lifelong learning. For would-be doctors, they must be prepared to meet the demands of higher education in science subjects. In the past, the educational system has largely been driven by success in examinations. These tend to reward memory and recall of factual information.

The medical curriculum is designed to provide a general medical education for all types of doctor and to serve as the foundation for later career specialization. The programme focuses on the development of clinical competence, usually beginning with laboratory-based clinical skills. Competence is then further developed during clinical components. There is an increasing emphasis on personal and professional development, including student choice and community-based medicine. An integrated approach is adopted with new information and skills introduced which link back to the elements covered earlier.

GENERAL CLINICAL TRAINING

In more recent years it has become the norm for all doctors to undergo a period of general professional training, with a year as a Pre-Registration House Officer (PRHO) and normally at least 2 years as a Senior House Officer.

General clinical training is aimed at building up the clinical experience of the doctor to prepare them for higher specialist training. Doctors in this period of training should be aiming to acquire and develop the attitudes, knowledge and skills to enable them ultimately to practise independently (see Box 5.1).

The pre-registration year is now seen as the final year of basic medical education. It has two purposes. It is to enable PRHOs to put into practice the key skills that they have learned and apply knowledge gained during

Box 5.1   Attributes of the independent medical practitioner

1. The ability to solve clinical and other problems in medical practice, which involves or requires:
   (a) an intellectual and temperamental ability to change, to face the unfamiliar and to adapt to change;
   (b) a capacity for individual, self-directed learning; and
   (c) reasoning and judgement in the application of knowledge to the analysis and interpretation of data, in defining the nature of a problem, and in planning and implementing a strategy to resolve it.
2. Possession of adequate knowledge and understanding of the general structure and function of the human body and workings of the mind, in health and disease, of their interaction and of the interaction between man and his physical and social environment. This requires:
   (a) knowledge of the physical, behavioural, epidemiological and clinical sciences upon which medicine depends;
   (b) understanding of the aetiology and natural history of diseases;
   (c) understanding of the impact of both psychological factors upon illness and of illness upon the patient and the patient's family;
   (d) understanding of the effects of childhood growth and of later ageing upon the individual, the family and the community; and
   (e) understanding of the social, cultural and environmental factors which contribute to health or illness, and the capacity of medicine to influence them.
3. Possession of consultation skills, which include:
   (a) skills in sensitive and effective communication with patients and their families, professional colleagues and local agencies, and the keeping of good medical records;
   (b) the clinical skills necessary to examine the patient's physical and mental state and to investigate appropriately;
   (c) the ability to exercise sound clinical judgement to analyse symptoms and physical signs in pathophysiological terms, to establish diagnoses, and to offer advice to the patient taking account of physical, psychological, social and cultural factors; and
   (d) understanding of the special needs of terminal care.
4. Acquisition of a high standard of knowledge and skills in the doctor's specialty, which include:
   (a) understanding of acute illness and of disabling and chronic diseases within that specialty, including their physical, mental and social implications, rehabilitation, pain relief, and the need for support and encouragement; and
   (b) relevant manual, biochemical, pharmacological, psychological, social and other interventions in acute and chronic illness.
5. Willingness and ability to deal with common medical emergencies and with other illness in an emergency.
6. The ability to contribute appropriately to the prevention of illness and the promotion of health, which involves:
   (a) understanding of the principles, methods and limitations of preventive medicine and health promotion;
   (b) understanding of the doctor's role in educating patients, families and communities, and in generally promoting good health; and
   (c) the ability to identify individuals at risk and to take appropriate action.
7. The ability to recognize and analyse ethical problems so as to enable patients, their families, society and the doctor to have proper regard to such problems in reaching decisions; this comprehends:
   (a) knowledge of the ethical standards and legal responsibilities of the medical profession;
   (b) understanding of the impact of medico-social legislation on medical practice; and
   (c) recognition of the influence upon his or her approach to ethical problems of the doctor's own personality and values.

Lifelong learning

8. The maintenance of attitudes and conduct appropriate to a high level of professional practice, which includes:
   (a) recognition that a blend of scientific and humanitarian approaches is required, involving a critical approach to learning, open-mindedness, compassion, and concern for the dignity of the patient and, where relevant, of the patient's family;
   (b) recognition that good medical practice depends on partnership between doctor and patient, based upon mutual understanding and trust; the doctor may give advice, but the patient must decide whether or not to accept it;
   (c) commitment to providing high quality care; awareness of the limitations of the doctor's own knowledge and of existing medical knowledge; recognition of the duty to keep up to date in the doctor's own specialist field and to be aware of developments in others; and
   (d) willingness to accept review, including self-audit, of the doctor's performance.

9. Mastery of the skills required to work within a team and, where appropriate, assume the responsibilities of team leader, which requires:
   (a) recognition of the need for the doctor to collaborate in prevention, diagnosis, treatment and management with other health care professionals and with patients themselves;
   (b) understanding and appreciation of the roles, responsibilities and skills of nurses and other health care workers; and
   (c) the ability to lead, guide and co-ordinate the work of others.

10. Acquisition of experience in administration and planning, including:
   (a) efficient management of the doctor's own time and professional activities;
   (b) appropriate use of diagnostic and therapeutic resources, and appreciation of the economic and practical constraints affecting the provision of health care; and
   (c) willingness to participate, as required, in the work of bodies which advise, plan and assist the development and administration of medical services, such as NHS authorities and trusts, Royal Colleges and Faculties, and professional associations.

11. Recognition of the opportunities and acceptance of the duty to contribute, when possible, to the advancement of medical knowledge and skill, which entails:
   (a) understanding of the contribution of research methods, and interpretation and application of others' research in the doctor's own specialty; and
   (b) willingness, when appropriate, to contribute to research in the doctor's specialist field, both personally and through encouraging participation by junior colleagues.

12. Recognition of the obligation to teach others, particularly doctors in training, which requires:
   (a) acceptance of responsibility for training junior colleagues in the specialty, and for teaching other doctors, medical students, and other health care professionals, when required;
   (b) recognition that teaching skills are not necessarily innate but can be learned, and willingness to acquire them; and
   (c) recognition that the example of the teacher is the most powerful influence upon the standards of conduct and practice of every trainee.

(Source: General Medical Council: *The Early Years*, 1998.)

undergraduate medical education. It is also to enable PRHOs to demonstrate that, on completing general clinical training, they are ready to accept with confidence the duties and responsibilities of a fully registered doctor and to begin training for specialist medical practice.

The pre-registration year is based on increasing responsibility for patient care, under the overall supervision of a fully trained specialist. The sort of

| Box 5.2 | Basic clinical skills |

- history taking
- clinical examination
- clinical testing
- diagnostic tests
- planning clinical management
- treatment
- review
- rehabilitation
- palliative care
- terminal care

basic clinical skills that should be evident in the performance of PRHOs are listed in Box 5.2.

At the present time there is little coherence or systematic approach to the Senior House Officer period of training, but reforms are currently being planned at the time of writing. It is likely that an approach based on the present approach to higher specialist training will be introduced. This period of basic training would be carried out within a series of programmes over a period of 2 or 3 years. The programmes would loosely cover medicine in general, surgery in general, general practice, mental illness in general, obstetrics and gynaecology, child health, anaesthesia, and pathology in general.

HIGHER SPECIALIST TRAINING

It is only relatively recently that higher training has become the norm in medical education, and even more recently that there has been the widespread acceptance of the notion of a commitment to a lifetime of continuing medical education and now continuing professional development. A basic professional qualification is no longer sufficient for a long-term occupation.

Higher specialist training aims to refine the generic skills acquired during general clinical training, and to develop specialist skills to equip doctors for specialist practice as consultants or general practitioners in the National Health Service.

Since the Calman reforms of specialist training (named after the then Chief Medical Officer, Sir Kenneth Calman), introduced in 1996 and 1997, entry to higher specialist training has been by competitive entry. For general practice, 1 year of training as a GP Registrar must be undertaken, together with relevant or prescribed hospital or other experience totalling a minimum of 3 years. There are concerns among many doctors and their specialist Royal Colleges that the time available for training is insufficient to gain the requisite breadth and depth of knowledge, skill or experience. Many trainees recognize that, even on the satisfactory completion of specialist training, they are ill equipped to take on the wide range of responsibilities normally associated with being a consultant in the NHS or a principal in general practice.

Lifelong learning

LIFELONG LEARNING

As the useful lifespan of knowledge gained declines, the need for continuing education becomes more urgent. It is now generally accepted that learning, professional development and growth continue throughout one's personal career, and indeed, the whole of one's lifetime. This is the concept of continuous lifelong learning (see Figure 5.1) as a process to keep abreast of change.

Lifelong learning is not merely about the acquisition of new skills as new technology or developments occur. It is also about refining the knowledge, skills and attitudes already possessed by the doctor.

The ability to keep up to date with the exponential explosion of knowledge is increasingly and severely tested. There are now over 25 000 biomedical journals published annually worldwide. Information is also available in many other modern media formats, such as on compact disc or tape. The explosion of information on the worldwide web is thought to be exponential. However, to be useful, information for health purposes has to be accurate and precise; junk must be identified and discarded. Librarians are the new knowledge managers.

Many doctors now combine many roles even in a single post. Not only may a doctor be a skilled clinician, he or she may also be a teacher, academic, researcher, manager. Indeed, doctors are increasingly opting to refine and deploy skills in these different areas at different stages of their professional life, leading to the concept of a portfolio career.

A portfolio career is one that may contain a number of jobs that are linked through professional development but not necessarily very directly. In the past, it was usual for a doctor, once appointed as a consultant to a particular post in a particular hospital, or as a partner in a particular general practice, to remain in that post until retirement. Now doctors change posts and practices in a search for perhaps a different clinical workload, or to pursue academic or managerial aspirations. One of the authors is now into his third

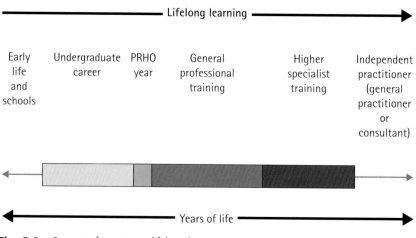

Fig. 5.1 Concept of continuous lifelong learning.

substantial career within medicine, once extremely unusual but now increasingly commonplace.

Learning needs have therefore changed over the years to reflect these developments, but the changes in health care currently underway and likely in the future present major educational challenges for doctors and others. The next generation of doctors will face an exploding volume of literature, the rapid introduction of new technologies, more demanding patients, and a much deeper focus on the quality and outcomes of medical care.

PRINCIPLES OF LEARNING

Training has been defined as a 'process of change occurring in a learner'.[4] Training programmes for postgraduates provide a form of higher education in which the learner is being trained to acquire skills more efficiently or more quickly than he or she would otherwise. Learning, on the other hand, is 'A relatively permanent change in behaviour that occurs as a result of practice or experience'.[5]

There are a number of general principles that are widely accepted as promoting learning. These include:

- Directing education and training towards meeting the needs of the learner; a learner is more easily able to learn, more likely to be involved and interested in the process, and more likely to succeed if he or she participates.
- Responsibility for learning must be shared; this recognizes that there may be learning through making mistakes.
- Learning by discovery: if, through intellectual involvement, struggling with the subject, and synthesizing for oneself the conclusions which are derived, the learner is able to discover a principle which it is intended should be learnt, there is more likely to be understanding and retention.
- Learning from peers: it is suggested that learners may gain more from teaching each other than from the traditional superior to inferior model. The effect of authority may be eliminated, and communication is often better.
- Reinforcement and repetition: all learning needs reinforcement; skills that are unpractised atrophy. Learners need opportunities to repeat the learning process, to practise the new skill or use the new knowledge. This may, of course, occur in clinical practice itself.
- An environment for learning: the appropriate atmosphere for learning to take place is an important matter of balance. A cosy atmosphere between trainer and trainee may be relaxed, but learning may not take place. Conversely, threat or too much anxiety or tension may inhibit the learning process.

In medicine, therefore, there is learning through immersion in clinical practice, both as a student and practitioner. There is the assumption of increasing responsibility. The apocryphal idea of 'see one; do one; teach one' may sometimes feel a little too close to the truth.

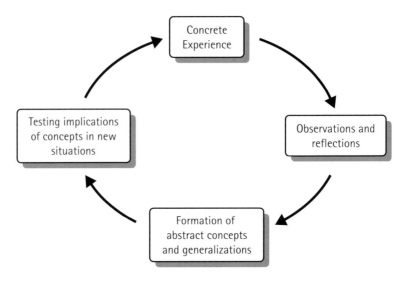

Fig. 5.2 Experiential learning. (After Kolb DA. On management and the learning process. In: Kolb DA, Rubin IN, McIntyre JM. *Organizational Psychology: A Book of Readings.* Englewood Cliffs, NJ: Prentice Hall, 1984.)

Of greater importance is the relevance of what is known as experiential learning (see Figure 5.2), based on the theoretical work of David Kolb. Kolb conceived the learning process as including four different but complementary kinds of abilities. In this model the learner reflects on a concrete experience, making observations about what went on. From such observations, and sometimes a number of experiences, the learner may then be able to derive a concept or generalization that ought to be applicable in other situations. The fourth part, of what is an iterative loop, consists of testing the theory in new and different situations.

THE SKILLS AND COMPETENCES REQUIRED IN DOCTORS

The practice of medicine requires skills in a wide range of domains. Many of these are generic and necessary for practice in almost every branch (see Box 5.3). Others are specialist, relating to narrowly defined areas of professional practice. Education and training, both undergraduate and postgraduate, are increasingly trying to instil and ensure competence in these skills. Medical Royal Colleges and faculties have been putting great effort into identifying these competencies. As yet, there is relatively little development of adequate methods of assessment, but these too are under development.

There is also a necessary and increasing focus on teamwork. The logic is simple: if doctors in future are to work in teams (and medical care will increasingly have to be delivered through teams and managed networks), then learning needs to take place in teams. One of the many recommendations

---

Box 5.3   Generic skills

Generic skills needed in clinical settings include:

- communication
- teamworking
- negotiation
- time management
- self-management
- priority setting
- knowledge management
- writing
- report writing
- clinical audit
- critical appraisal

---

from the Bristol inquiry proposed a common undergraduate foundation first year of training. This approach and others are being actively developed by the Workforce Development Confederations, who now have responsibility for all aspects of health professional development, education and training.

However, the shift of focus, particularly among the public and bodies responsible for regulation of the profession, is away from assessment of competency (the ability to be able to do things) towards assessment of performance, whether or not skills are appropriately and effectively applied in real life practice.

Although the apprenticeship model of training still largely prevails, other approaches are available to help the perhaps bewildered undergraduate or doctor move effectively along the lifelong learning spectrum.

There are now a number of validated tools for self-assessment available that help the learner identify their own learning and development needs. The steady progress in equipping trainers to better identify training needs is leading particularly to the steady application of sound educational processes during undergraduate and postgraduate medical training. Trainers are encouraging the application of the Kolb model of learning.

APPRAISAL AND FEEDBACK ON PERFORMANCE

Appraisal must now be undertaken at least annually by all NHS professional staff. It has been commonplace in higher specialist training, introduced as part of the Calman reforms to specialist training, and is a routine part of the undergraduate medical curriculum.

Appraisal has two principal purposes: it is intended to move the learner in terms of the ability to do the job better (to make care more efficient, in terms of doing things right, as well as effective, i.e. doing the right things), and to help the learner achieve what they want to achieve in the future in their career.

There are a number of particular features associated with effective appraisal:

- Confidentiality: conventionally, the process involved is confidential to appraiser and appraisee, although there may be, and now often needs to be, a more widely shared output.
- Training: both appraiser and appraisee should be trained.
- Preparation: both appraiser and appraisee need to prepare for an appraisal meeting.
- The appraisee's perspective: the reflection of the appraisee or trainee is central. Experience shows that most people are often more self-critical than their trainer or appraiser may be.
- The appraiser's perspective: the appraiser then shares his or her perspective. This should be couched in constructive terms, whether positive or negative, and should focus on behaviours displayed by the person being appraised. Indeed the whole focus is intended to be positive and developmental.
- An agreed outcome: there should be a written statement at the end of an appraisal that is agreed by appraisee and appraiser. This may reflect strengths and weaknesses, and plans for further action, including training, experience or other career development. This output may need to be shared as evidence contributing to assessment of performance.

There is a trend towards what can be called 360° appraisal. It is unlikely that an appraiser can know or have experience of all aspects of the trainee's work. Feedback from whatever source has always been a potential contributor to learning and development. Perceptions can be dismissed as being merely subjective, but perceptions are sometimes as close as we can get to reality. Seeking the views of others, particularly other health professionals (consultants, nursing staff), and possibly even peers and patients helps to provide a broader range of evidence for views expressed and examples of effective (and less effective) behaviours. Sometimes this can be achieved by participation, although appraisal rarely involves more than one or two appraisers. Validated questionnaires also exist. It is the idea of seeking feedback from superiors, as well as peers and those more junior colleagues, that gives rise to the notion of '360°' appraisal.

One crucial outcome of appraisal should be a personal development plan. This should identify areas of experience or skills for further development, how this is to be achieved, by when, and how success will be judged (see Boxes 5.4 and 5.5).

An important potential spin-off from appraisal concerns activities, such as teaching and training, that have hitherto often remained hidden. Appraisal should make both the time and the effectiveness of such work much more explicit. This makes such work more accessible for recognition purposes, and where deficiencies – such as the availability of time with competing pressures – impinge on effectiveness or even meeting such a fundamental responsibility.

The personal development or learning plan must be primarily derived from self-motivation. It must be realistic and achievable within a specified timescale. It should be agreed between the appraiser and appraisee. Elements

Box 5.4   An example of a personal development plan (1)

What do I need to learn?
To communicate effectively with patients from all walks of life

How did I identify this need?
Self-diagnosis
Discussion with educational supervisor
Observations from colleagues and patients

How will I learn it?
Attend a communications skills course
Observation of acknowledged good communicators
Asking patients what they have understood after I have given an explanation
Ask nurses for feedback
Video consultations

What resources do I need?
Information about communication skills course
An educational supervisor who is skilled in communication
Opportunities to work with good communicators and get feedback from them
Nurses and others who are willing and able to give good quality feedback
Time
Funding for the course

How long will this take?
Identifying, enrolling for and undergoing a course may take 6 months
Should be some improvement within 6 months, but may take longer

How will I measure when I have learned it?
I will notice that I put some communication skills into practice
I will find it easier to understand other people's points of view
Patients will have understood what I have said
The nurses and doctors with whom I work will give positive feedback

Reflections on each element:
What did I learn?
How did I learn it?
Which factors helped me to learn?
What changed as a result?

Box 5.5   An example of a personal development plan (2)

Background: this trainee found it difficult to site epidurals in obstetric patients. He did several dural taps, and lost confidence in his abilities.

What do I need to learn?
To site epidural catheters and achieve a successful epidural block in obstetric patients

How will I learn it?
Practise with a model
Regain confidence by siting epidurals in non-obstetric patients
Close observation of the technique used by a number of trainers
Trainers giving precise description of the technical aspects of the procedure as they site
    epidurals
Being observed siting epidurals
Reflection about the circumstances in which difficulties occur (e.g. is it identifying the loss
    of resistance, threading the catheter, etc?)

What resources do I need?
The opportunity to do epidurals in non-pregnant patients
Access to a model
The opportunity to work with several trainers
The opportunity to be observed, and to have detailed discussions with trainers

How long will this take?
About 25 epidurals probably needed, so depends on the frequency of opportunities to work

How will I measure when I have learned it?
I will feel confident
Few (ideally no) dural taps
Trainers happy to let me work without direct supervision

Reflections on each element:
What did I learn?
How did I learn it?
Which factors helped me to learn?
What changed as a result?

that it contains should either be aimed at helping the person do their job better or helping them achieve career objectives some time in the future (see Box 5.6).

Personal continuing professional development should motivate the individual and stimulate behaviour change in priority areas of professional practice that will enhance (directly or indirectly) the delivery of effective health care.

Box 5.6   The requirement of objectives

Personal objectives should be SMART:

- S   pecific
- M   easurable
- A   chievable
- R   ealistic
- T   imetabled

MENTORING

One route to helping people achieve their full potential is through mentoring. Mentoring means different things in different contexts. A mentor has been described as a role model, a guide, a tutor, a coach, or a confidant.[6] Conventionally, mentors are often 8–15 years senior. Mentors are not usually the person's immediate boss, because the two roles can conflict. Many people choose mentors informally without any preconceived idea of their suitability or skills. Mentors are best when able to assist from a neutral perspective, i.e. they should not be a superior or in a line management position with regard to the mentee. The basis of ad hoc selection is usually respect for and knowledge of the individual. However, to achieve success, the possession of skills is likely to help. Trained mentors should have the skills and ability to help clarify, probe and challenge their mentees, since their role is to assist the person in the management of changes as they are perceived to affect them. They also help by assisting the mentee in identifying possible strategies, analysing and deciding which are most appropriate, and devising plans for achieving them.

Mentoring can be used to advantage in inducting newcomers efficiently into the organization. They are able to help with organizational problems as well as personal development, and this can increase motivation and job satisfaction. A properly organized scheme of mentoring can therefore be an inexpensive and efficient way of developing people.

Whilst individual competence and performance are crucial in relation to doctors caring for patients, increasing attention is being given to the organization. It is considered that over three quarters of significant events occurring in the NHS are due to system failures. Systems aspects of clinical governance are dealt with elsewhere in this book.

CONTINUING PROFESSIONAL DEVELOPMENT

It is worth spending a moment reflecting on the evolution of postgraduate courses into continuing medical education, through continuing professional development, into what we now need to think of as lifelong learning.

In the early years after the foundation of the NHS in 1948, hospital postgraduate medical centres were where general practitioners had the opportunity, usually at a fixed weekday lunchtime or occasionally during an evening session, to meet with local consultants who would be presenting lectures. The remnants of this history can still be seen in a variety of Wednesday or Thursday lunchtime lecture programmes.

With the realization that the pace of development of medical knowledge was accelerating, the notion of continuing medical education evolved. This recognized the need to keep up to date. The media for this transposition of knowledge remained narrow, confined essentially to a comparatively small number of medical journals, such as the *Lancet* and the *British Medical Journal*, and the traditional lecture, with frequent occurrences of sessions entitled 'Recent advances in … '.

At the present time things have moved towards continuing professional development (CPD). Royal Colleges and faculties have recognized the need to sustain and maintain knowledge and skills and almost all now require their members to undergo a minimum prescribed package each year. Continuing professional development is purposeful, systematic activity by individuals, and possibly their organizations, to maintain and develop the knowledge, skills and attributes which are needed for effective professional practice. CPD is a professional obligation for all doctors in the UK. The defined package, different for each college or faculty, is a minimum and some make certain privileges, such as being a trainer or a College visitor, conditional upon maintenance of a CPD record.

Now linked with other developments, such as appraisal, is the fundamental precept that one never stops learning and developing; adaptive change to thrive in a modern world. This is lifelong learning, built on the basic self-questioning approach and search for what will help one do the job better.

The broadening out of approaches to continuing learning in the field of medicine has been led by the pioneering work to develop vocational training for general practice. In the early 1970s the limitations of the traditional lecture were recognized, in that they did not meet the needs of modern general practitioners. Using the paradigm of defining aims for training, applying relevant methods (depending on the aims), coupled with assessment, vocational training forged ahead. One-to-one tutorials, seminars and small group work became highly developed. Once analysis of the consultation was made possible, the consequent taxonomy allowed teaching approaches to be developed. This work on the consultation, particularly with respect to aspects of communication with the patient through the whole range of the traditional approach to medicine (diagnosis and hypothesis testing, management planning and implementation, review and reassessment) remains the envy of many other specialties.

Teaching and learning need to use methods that are most appropriate to the aims and objectives of what is to be learnt. Examples of educational interventions or approaches are shown in Box 5.7. A brief analysis of some of the available methods can be seen in Box 5.8.

Box 5.7   Some educational interventions or approaches

Formal teaching:	Lectures and presentations
	Case presentations
	Specific curriculum sessions
	Small group tutorials
Opportunistic teaching:	Grand rounds/ward rounds
	Hand-over
	Clinics
	'Special' clinics
Planned supervision:	For example, anaesthetic or surgical teaching list
	Consultant and trainee seeing patient together
	Physician's clinic
	Planned formal one to one
Independent practice:	Supervised reflective graded responsibility
Hand-over/debrief	Clinical
	Generic
	Post-take ward round

Peer learning
e-learning
Distance learning
Tele-conferencing
Teaching others
Team learning
Journal clubs
Departmental meetings
Clinical audit
Critical incident reviews/significant event analysis

Simulations:	Actors
	Computers
	3-D
	Skills laboratories
'SWOT' analysis	Strenghts, Weaknesses, Opportunities, Threats

Box 5.8 Strengths and weaknesses of some different educational approaches

Teaching and learning modality	Strengths	Weaknesses	Notes
Lectures	• Impart knowledge to comparatively large numbers • Well used so skills relatively widely dispersed • High quality lecturers can enthuse and inspire	• Often mediocre skills possessed by lecturers • Disproportionate time spent preparing • Largely about transmission of facts • Only small proportion of facts may be learned or recalled	• Costly facilities required (e.g. theatre, audio-visual equipment) • Helped by handouts
Seminars or workshop groups	• May be more inclusive and participative • Should involve preparation and participation of all • Relevance tends to be higher	• Works best with small numbers • Groups need to work together and evolve for maximum functionality and effectiveness • Leader or facilitator needs to be highly skilled and experienced	• Particularly useful for generating new ideas, gaining commitment or problem solving
Tutorials	• One to one • May capitalize on opportunities	• Tutor needs to be skilled	• Can be 'brief bites' of learning
Private study	• Arguably, should be most learner-centred • Minimum facilities required	• Learner needs to be highly motivated	
Shadowing	• Provides valuable insights	• Time-consuming • Needs time for reflection	• Requires careful planning, briefing and debriefing
Action learning	• Used for problem solving, and changing individuals, teams and organizations	• More effective with a trained facilitator • Needs discipline	
Locums/acting up	• Qualitatively and quantitatively different experience	• Only a limited time can count to training	• Requires careful planning, briefing and debriefing
Formal courses and higher degrees	• Structured • Explicit objectives and methods • Lead to recognized qualification	• Costly in time and funding • Needs high learner commitment and motivation • Structure and content predetermined, so may not be tailored to learner's needs	

REVALIDATION

Another major reformist plank is revalidation by the General Medical Council. No longer will registration after satisfactory completion of the pre-registration house year be sufficient to maintain the right to professional practice (unless found guilty of serious professional misconduct). Instead revalidation every 5 years will be required.

Revalidation will be achieved through aggregation of a portfolio of evidence gained over each 5-year period relating to professional practice in the specific job that the doctor does, whatever its content or specialty. Local revalidation panels, which will include lay representatives, will make decisions on revalidation or, in the case of those in whom doubts arise, referral to the GMC for more rigorous and detailed assessment under the GMC performance procedures.

Other routes for assessment or referral can be as a result of an assessment by the Commission for Health Audit and Inspection, or via the National Clinical Assessment Authority (see Chapter 1).

CONCLUSION

Patients expect their doctors and dentists to be knowledgeable and skilled, and trust them to provide the highest standards of care. The NHS has a responsibility to ensure that its doctors are trained and develop the necessary skills and competences to practise medicine and meet the health care needs of patients. Doctors have a responsibility to maintain and develop these skills throughout their professional lives.

REFERENCES

1. General Medical Council. *Good Medical Practice*. London: General Medical Council, 1998.
2. Reid MA, Barrington H. *Training Interventions: Managing Employee Development*. London: Institute of Personnel and Development, 1994.
3. Report of the Committee of Inquiry into the Regulation of the Medical Profession. London: HMSO, 1975 (Cmd 6018).
4. Bass BM, Vaughan JA. *Training in Industry – The Management of Learning*. London: Tavistock Publications, 1966.
5. Watkins J, Drury L, Preddy D. *From Evolution to Revolution: The Pressures on Professional Life in the 1990s*. University of Bristol, 1992.
6. Clutterbuck D. *Everyone Needs a Mentor*. London: Institute of Personnel Management, 1991.

Monitoring quality of care: reducing errors and improving standards

6

'But for the grace of God, there goes John Bradford.'

John Bradford, 1542

Inevitably we have a biased view of our own performance. Anecdotal experience with individual patients can lead us to remember the good and forget the bad. In order to improve our self-assessment and learning from history, we need open and systematic methods to inform us. This chapter covers clinical audit and risk management methods that aim to improve quality of care and reduce errors. It covers the following topics:

- Medical errors and risk management
- Prescribing errors
- Clinical audit
- National confidential enquiries
- Control charts.

REDUCING MEDICAL ERRORS AND IMPROVING PATIENT SAFETY

Until recently, medical errors or adverse events have been a taboo subject for doctors. A culture of blame and shame has prevented any rational attempt to learn from our failures and prevent recurrences. Doctors have for too long been considered as infallible and when mistakes do happen there has been nowhere for them to turn for support or discussion. Thus the doctor becomes isolated in his guilt and defensiveness and the patient becomes angry at the lack of honesty.

When patients are asked why they are pursuing complaints and litigation, the primary motivation is not money or revenge; it is to ensure that the same mistake does not happen to other patients. Doctors and health professionals share this motivation, although the threat of litigation and disciplinary procedures stifles a culture of openness and learning.

It is estimated that about 10% of inpatient episodes will lead to adverse events, half of which are preventable. For the whole NHS this translates as nearly a million admissions every year leading to adverse mistakes, at a potential cost of up to £2 billion from extended hospital admissions. Common errors include prescribing errors – wrong drug, wrong dose (e.g. adult dose given to a child), wrong administration (e.g. intravenous cytotoxic drugs given intrathecally); communication failures; delays in diagnosis.

Previous approaches to human error have focused on individuals and blamed their actions on carelessness, tiredness, inattention or negligence. Fellow professionals breathe a sigh of relief and quote John Bradford. This is the easy approach, with someone identified to be the fall guy. However, even the best doctors make mistakes, and errors are not random events, but follow the same patterns. The same adverse events happen over and over again, not only in other hospitals, but also in the same hospital over time.

Individual factors are an important part of clinical practice; however, they are only one component. When an adverse mistake occurs, the individual factor may just be the last, but most visible link in a rusting chain of errors that owes more to the context or system within which the health professional is working. These may include poor teamwork and communication, staff shortages, time pressures, lack of experience or inadequate equipment. To err is to be human, and adverse events will always occur. However, we can reduce their frequency by learning from them and putting into place defences in the system that will reduce the risk of individual mistakes (Box 6.1).

Medical errors: The correct leg

It was another busy Monday morning. It was a whole day theatre day and my boss and I had been going round to see all the patients beforehand.

The last patient we saw was a woman who was due to have an operation on her. Achilles tendon. She turned round and lay prone as we examined her. Then we put a big black arrow on her calf.

After that, we returned to theatre and began operating. It is our practice to recheck every patient routinely before they are anaesthetised.

After finishing the second case, we went to the anaesthetic room to check our next patient, who was the woman with the tendon problem. We noticed that she had an arrow on the front of her right leg, although she was due to have an operation on the left one. We were embarrassed and did not know what to say. But then we realised that she also had an arrow on her left calf.

For a few minutes we did not realise what had happened. Then it occurred to us that after we had put the arrow on her left calf, she had crossed her left leg over the right one and had made an impression of this arrow on the front of her right leg. Hence the arrow on both legs.

Finally, the confusion was resolved and we operated on the correct leg. We learnt an important lesson – that one should always mark the operation site in a way that is not going to lead to ambiguity.

Subhasish Deb *clinical research fellow in orthopaedics,*
John Aldridge *consultant orthopaedic surgeon, Coventry*

(Reproduced with permission from: *BMJ* 2001; **322**: 602.)

Box 6.1   The terrible tale of intrathecal injections – changing the system

Between 1985 and 2001 there have been 14 cases where junior doctors have injected intrathecal vincristine (or other vinca alkaloids) by mistake. The drugs are important in the treatment of leukaemia, but must be given intravenously. Intrathecal injection results in death or paralysis.

These mistakes have received a lot of medical and public attention. On several occasions the junior doctors have been charged with manslaughter. Despite such awareness of the devastating consequences of such mistakes, they continue because we are only human, and humans err. In some cases the doctors were unfamiliar or untrained. In others the drug tray contained both intravenous and intrathecal drugs – a recipe for disaster. In other cases again, on-call fatigue or patients being treated on outlying wards contributed to the fatal mistakes.

Safeguards have been used to try and prevent these tragedies. For example, ensuring that cytoxic drugs are given only by specially trained staff, using clear warnings, giving intrathecal drugs only in operating theatres and giving them alone rather than with other drugs. However, it is likely that repeat mistakes will occur until we come up with a foolproof method of ensuring that intravenous drugs cannot be given intrathecally. The solution probably lies in designing unique administration systems. A similar solution in anaesthetics has prevented deaths caused by mixing up nitrous oxide and oxygen tanks, as connections are no longer compatible.

REDUCING ERRORS

The methods and proposals for reducing medical errors have drawn heavily on approaches used in other sectors with more experience, particularly the airline industry. Like the health care industry, the airline industry is extremely complex and every error is potentially lethal. However, if the airline industry had a similar error rate to the health care industry then we would have aircraft falling out of the sky all over the place. Other sectors such as nuclear power plants also provide examples for risk management. A model that both these industries use is that of the 'Swiss cheese' (Figure 6.1), with different layers of defences preventing errors from happening. However, each of these layers can develop holes, and if these holes line up then errors can occur. In medicine, there can be dangerously few protective slices of cheese and this can cause disaster.

The approach that the airline industry took to reduce errors was to ensure that every mistake, and more importantly, every near miss was identified and reported. There will be tens and hundreds of near misses for every reported error, and so these are important to identify and to rectify before they end up as mistakes.

Reporting systems are integral to working practices in the industry and great emphasis is placed on a willingness to learn from incidents rather than attach blame. In contrast, the health service has patchy and haphazard reporting systems, with no standardized definitions for adverse events and a culture of guilt and cover-up.

In 2000/2001, the Chief Medical Officer's report *An organisation with a memory* and subsequent implementation paper *Building a safer NHS* identified barriers to organizational learning (Box 6.2) and outlined a series of steps to

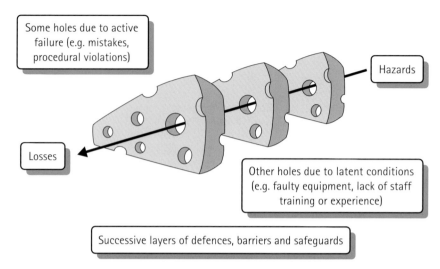

Fig. 6.1 The 'Swiss cheese' model of accident causation.

Box 6.2   Barriers to organizational learning

- An undue focus on the immediate event rather than on the root cause(s) of problems
- Latching onto one superficial cause or learning point to the exclusion of more fundamental but sometimes less obvious lessons
- Rigidity of core beliefs, values and assumptions, which may develop over time – learning is resisted if it contradicts these
- Lack of corporate responsibility – it may be difficult, for example, to put into practice solutions which are sufficiently far-reaching
- Ineffective communication and other information difficulties – including failure to disseminate information which is readily available
- An incremental approach to issues of risk – attempting to resolve problems through tinkering rather than tackling more fundamental change
- Pride in organizational and individual expertise can lead to denial and to a disregard of external sources of warning – particularly if a bearer of bad news lacks legitimacy in the eyes of the individuals, teams or organizations in question
- A tendency towards scapegoating and finding individuals to blame – rather than acknowledging and addressing deep-rooted organizational problems
- The difficulties faced by people in 'making sense' of complex events is compounded by changes among key personnel within organizations and teams
- Human alliances lead people to 'forgive' other team members their mistakes and act defensively against ideas from outside the team
- People are often unwilling to learn from negative events, even when it would be to their advantage
- Contradictory imperatives – for example, communication versus confidentiality
- High stress and low job satisfaction can have adverse effects on quality and can also engender a resistance to change
- Inability to recognize the financial costs of failure, thus losing a powerful incentive for organizations to change

(Source: Department of Health: *An Organization with a Memory*. London: The Stationery Office, 2000.)

improve learning from mistakes. Central to the recommendations is the establishment of a mandatory system in the NHS for the reporting and learning from errors and adverse events. This system will:

- Be based on sound and confidential local reporting systems.
- Agree definitions and establish reliable categorization and reporting of:
  - adverse health care incidents: an event or omission arising during clinical care and causing physical or psychological injury to the patient.
  - health care near misses: a situation in which an event or omission arising during clinical care fails to develop further and injury to the patient is prevented.
- Set out a minimum dataset for adverse events and near misses which will include:
  - what happened?
  - where and when did it happen?
  - how and why did it happen?
  - what action was taken and what impact did the event have?
  - what factors could have reduced the impact of the event?
- Standardize the reporting format for all events using an accurately maintained electronic database.
- Ensure clear and accessible channels for reporting by NHS staff, organizations, patients and other agencies (e.g. NHS Complaints, Commission for Health Improvement, Medical Devices Agency and Medicines Control Agency).
- Analyse reports to identify common factors and give feedback to clinical staff constructively (Table 6.1). This includes *root cause analysis* to find out why an event happened, what factors were important and what improvements could be made to reduce future risk to patients.

Reporting, analysis and feedback will occur through a combination of local systems and a national organisation, the National Patient Safety Agency (NPSA). This is a new independent body (website: http://www.npsa.org.uk/index2.htm), which was established as a special health authority on 2 July 2001. The NPSA will record adverse events and near misses. This agency will collate and analyse reports from across the NHS. These reports will be reviewed regularly with analysis of patterns and trends. As well as developing solutions to risk, the NPSA will be responsible for monitoring the impact of these solutions over time (Box 6.3).

Box 6.3 Four national targets for the NHS to reduce risk to patients

1. To reduce to zero the number of patients dying or injured by maladministration of spinal injections by the end of 2001.
2. To reduce by 25% the number of instances of harm in the field of obstetrics and gynaecology which result in litigation by the end of 2005.
3. To reduce by 40% the number of serious errors in the use of prescribed drugs by the end of 2005.
4. To reduce to zero the number of suicides by mental health patients as a result of hanging from non-collapsible bed or shower rails on wards by March 2002.

Table 6.1   A new approach to responding to adverse events in the NHS

Past	Future
Fear of reprisals common	Generally blame-free reporting policy
Individuals scapegoated	Individuals held to account where justified
Disparate adverse event databases	All databases coordinated
Staff do not always hear the outcome of an investigation	Regular feedback to front-line staff
Individual training dominant	Team-based training common
Attention focuses on individual error	Systems approach to identifying hazards and prevention
Lack of awareness of risk management	General risk management awareness training provided
Short-term fixing of problems	Emphasis on sustaining risk reduction
Manipulative use of data	Conscientious use of data
Many adverse events regarded as isolated 'one-offs'	Potential for replication of similar adverse events recognized
Lessons from adverse events seen as primarily for the service or team concerned	Recognition that lessons learned may be relevant to others
Passive learning	Active learning

(Source: Department of Health: An *Organisation with a Memory*. London: The Stationery Office, 2000.)

National systems are the easy part of any effort to reduce adverse events. They will only work if clinicians use them for reporting adverse events and near misses and have a willingness to learn from them. For this to happen then the culture is crucial; it must be open and blame-free, without fear of retribution. Changing culture is the tricky part, and this will take time and effective leadership within health organizations. One of the major barriers to a supportive and blame-free culture is the fact that the press and the general public want the naming and shaming of bad doctors. Good medical leadership and public education will be required to emphasize the reality that all doctors make mistakes and there is much to learn from these mistakes. This is a long way from disciplinary issues of poor performance and incompetence that concern us all.

The action needed to reduce future errors will come from the analysis and feedback. This may vary from ensuring that resuscitation trolleys are kept in a standard location on the ward, with standard layouts, to making sure that inexperienced doctors do not undertake new procedures without adequate supervision. Common development areas include:

- Better training and supervision with improved availability of senior support in order to reduce incorrect diagnoses and inappropriate clinical management.

- Better communication and timely delivery of information, particularly during hand-overs or transfers of patient care, e.g. between shifts or on discharge.
- Clinical guidelines or checklists to remind clinicians about correct procedures and treatment.
- Simplified systems to reduce confusion and options for error, for example, in reducing unnecessary paperwork or equipment.
- Standardized procedures to reduce unnecessary variation in clinical practices, drugs or equipment.
- Safer equipment to limit equipment error.
- Better information recorded in clinical notes to ensure all staff are kept up to date, and more importantly, for patients themselves to ensure that they understand and are fully informed.

Steps to error reduction in a clinical department

1. Agree a designated clinical risk lead in the department who is responsible for overseeing the reporting and managing of adverse events and near misses.
2. Raise awareness in the department about the importance of learning from mistakes and having systems for error reporting.
3. Sit down together to assess potential risks and ensure staff know how to report adverse patient incidents (adverse events and near misses).
4. Agree a list of trigger incidents that should form part of the reporting systems (Table 6.2) and ensure all staff are aware of what incidents should be reported.
5. Promote accurate and comprehensive reporting. Ongoing reinforcement will help to achieve wider involvement.
6. Collate all reported incidents onto a risk management database with minimum dataset details about the incident, how it happened, why it happened, what impact it had and how this could have been minimized.
7. Grade incidents according to seriousness and likelihood of recurrence. All serious incidents should be reported immediately to the designated lead and where necessary to external agencies, e.g. Department of Health, Health and Safety Executive.
8. Analyse and review summaries of reports on a monthly basis. Investigate incidents according to seriousness (Boxes 6.4 and 6.5).
9. Discuss the results at monthly departmental clinical governance meetings to learn and disseminate lessons.
10. Agree action to reduce common and potentially serious incidents.
11. Implement and monitor improvement strategies.

Barriers to comprehensive and accurate reporting, such as the paperwork involved, lack of time or anxiety over how the reports will be used, should be acknowledged and addressed. Training, supportive and blame-free feedback and demonstrable action to improve care are all important aspects of ensuring that staff regularly report events.

Table 6.2   Clinical risk incidents

Obstetrics	Ophthalmology
Failed ventouse/forceps	Operation on the wrong eye
Cord prolapse/shoulder dystocia	Wrong operation on correct eye
Stillbirth/neonatal death	Missing case notes at surgery
3rd/4th degree tear	Penetration or perforation of globe during peri-ocular injection
Low Apgar <4 at 5 minutes	Expulsive haemorrhage during surgery
Neonatal injury or convulsions	Endophthalmitis following surgery
Meconium aspiration	Patient collapse requiring resuscitation during surgery
Very low birth weight <900 g	Death
Unanticipated admission to SCBU	'Open' category for incidents causing concern among staff for whatever reason
Drug error	Unplanned return to the operating theatre within 28 days for surgery for treatment of the same eye
High dependency care	Unplanned readmission to an eye unit within 28 days of surgery for treatment of the same eye
Return to theatre	Unplanned transfer or referral of patients to other ophthalmic units within 28 days of surgery

---

Box 6.4   Incident investigation and root cause analysis

The degree of investigation of reported incidents will be limited by constraints of time and resources. Efforts should be concentrated on serious incidents, with investigation of less serious incidents carried out on aggregated information. Investigations should aim to explore why the incident happened and what the underlying causes were. Evidence can be collected from *case note review, interviews with staff or direct observation* of procedures or equipment. Recommendations to prevent recurrence should be made and an improvement plan agreed and implemented.

Root cause analysis should be undertaken for all serious incidents and will identify underlying causes and system failures and explain their potential role in the event. A team of appropriate staff with senior management support is assigned to investigate contributing factors. These may be the obvious and immediate causes related to the patient or professional, or the more important underlying and root causes related to the systems and organizations. The root cause analysis should focus on opportunities to improve systems, plan how these opportunities can be addressed and explain who will implement the plan, the timescale and how change will be measured.

Reporting of adverse events will always be incomplete. The only way to ensure that all potential adverse events are recorded would be to review every set of case notes, and while this does occur in some North American hospitals, it is unlikely ever to be affordable in the NHS. However, electronic patient records may allow some routine monitoring in the future.

Box 6.5   Learning from catastrophe – root cause analysis

A 45-year-old man was admitted at 8 pm with an abscess on his left thigh. One of the two surgical house officers on call was off sick and so to help out, the surgical SHO clerked the patient in A&E. He noted in the history that the patient had a penicillin allergy, having had stridor following one oral dose when younger. No case notes were requested and the history remained on a loose sheet.

The patient was admitted to the ward where he was seen during an evening ward round. None of the staff on the round had been involved in his admission. The on-call theatre was busy so a drainage operation was postponed until morning. The consultant asked for the patient to be written up for some IV Magnapen to prevent any development of septicaemia in the interim.

The house officer wrote up the Magnapen on the chart, and at the evening drug round a ward nurse, not connecting Magnapen with penicillin, gave his first IV dose. The man arrested and, despite attempts at resuscitation, died.

Following this tragedy a root cause analysis was undertaken to determine the lessons to be learnt to prevent recurrence. The following 'holes' in the system were identified:

- The failure to obtain case notes that had the pencillin allergy clearly documented
- The lack of safety net for medical staff cover when the house officer went off sick
- The omission of clerking on the ward and subsequent unfamiliarity of patient with staff
- The lack of theatre time to undertake the operation that evening
- A confusing variety of drug charts, some (including the patient's) with no section for recording allergy
- Unfamiliarity with the drug trade name and its connection with penicillin
- Lack of support for the patient's family and for staff involved following the tragedy.

Changes were subsequently implemented to standardize drug charts and drug stocks, provide better locum cover, availability of case notes and staff and family support. Crucially, no disciplinary action was taken against the staff involved.

Reports of risk incident and adverse events should be supplemented with other information and surveillance (Figure 6.2). These include the following aspects.

Complaints and claims (see Chapter 8): these form an essential part of improving care, as they represent adverse events that are reported by the patient rather than the professional. It is important that the complaints and claims department works closely with the clinical risk lead for the department to ensure that all reports are collated and fed back to staff so that lessons can be learnt and future reports prevented.

Critical incident surveillance: it may be impossible to review every set of case notes, but reviewing high risk patients can be informative and can pick up adverse events that have not been detected or recorded. For example, in obstetrics, reviewing the notes of babies admitted to special care units may detect causative factors such as abnormal CTG readings or unrecognized pyrexia in the mother.

Clinical incident panels: a panel of staff from the department who screen all the reported adverse events and identify where there is concern over the quality of care provided or the clinical outcome.

Risk assessment: a more proactive approach to identifying potential risk. This involves collating standards and guidelines (such as CNST, controls assurance) for a department and then going round to staff and asking them

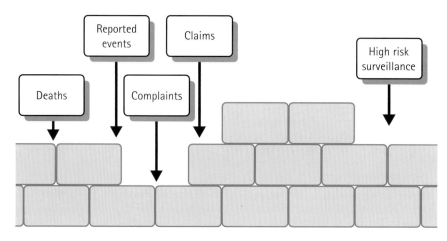

Fig. 6.2 A strong foundation. Sources of information for monitoring risk and errors.

if these are implemented in practice, if the environment is appropriate and where there are gaps in practice. For example, a risk assessment exercise may identify that locum staff are not receiving inductions, or that there is not sufficient training in CPR, or that old equipment needs replacement. Such assessment results can then contribute to a register for risk reports.

Learning from events in other organizations: hospitals and primary care trusts do not need to wait for a serious adverse event to occur that has already happened elsewhere. Such events should prompt an internal review to determine 'if it could happen here' and if so what steps can be taken to reduce the risk of such an occurrence (see Box 6.6).

Box 6.6   Reducing X-ray mistakes

An Accident and Emergency Department found that it had a 5% rate of missed fractures and foreign body detection on emergency films. When they reviewed the process of radiology reporting, they found that it varied depending on the day and the time of day, with radiologists reporting films during normal working hours, and A&E doctors reporting films out of hours and at weekends.

The high rate of missed abnormalities prompted a review of the reporting system, with all X-rays reported by A&E doctors and then also reported by radiologists within 12 hours. Any differences in reports were then reviewed at a combined monthly meeting. Within 1 month of introduction of the revised system, the rate of missed abnormalities had fallen to 2%.

PRESCRIBING ERRORS

In an average hospital, doctors will prescribe between 1 and 2 million drugs per year and nurses will administer approximately 30 million doses of medication. Even a low rate of prescribing errors will lead to large numbers of potential adverse events, and current evidence suggests that prescribing

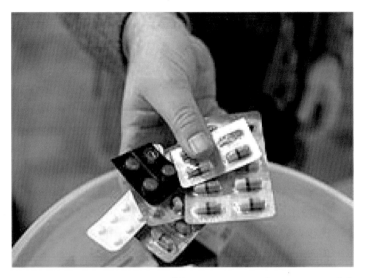

Fig. 6.3 Getting it right ... being aware of the common prescribing errors can help to avoid mistakes being made.

errors are common. Surveys have suggested that over 10% of prescriptions contain errors, some of them potentially fatal.

Prescribing errors account for up to 25% of litigation claims in medical practice. Review of these claims shows how the same mistakes are made over and over again, and yet the common lessons underlying them are rarely learnt outside the courtroom.

1. *Write clearly.* Illegible writing may provide a light-hearted caricature of doctors, but in these days of enormous variety and complexity of prescribing choices, there is no room for uncertainty. Prescriptions must clearly state the drug, dose and frequency.
2. *Obtain an accurate drug history.* Drug histories can be difficult to obtain, with patients admitted to hospital in various states of anxiety, disorientation, reduced consciousness, intoxication or dementia. Omitting drugs can be just as important as prescribing drugs, for example, patients on anti-convulsants, anti-arrhythmics or insulin.
3. *Make sure the dose is correct.* Sometimes this is due to carelessness, with doses being calculated on the basis of 'that seems about right'. With children this can lead to serious overdoses, with doses calculated to the wrong decimal point, or on the basis of mg/kg/day rather than mg/kg/dose.
4. *Make sure the timing of dose is correct.* Some drugs such as statins may be given once daily, but should also be given at night. Some antibiotics are given TDS, some QDS. Some drugs such as methotrexate for arthritis or psoriasis are given once a week, yet commonly end up written down as once a day, leading to serious overdoses.

5. *Stop drugs* that are no longer needed such as postoperative IV antibiotics. *Start drugs* that should be given, such as heparin for thromboprophylaxis.
6. *Check contra-indications* and drug interactions. Warn the patient of possible side effects.
7. *Check with the patient.* Ask about drug allergies before prescribing. Check with the patient before dispensing.
8. *Check with a colleague* before dispensing unusual drugs or doses.
9. Make sure you are prescribing the *right drug for the right patient.* Common errors include prescribing drugs to the wrong patient.

The overall lesson is simple: don't guess – look it up or ask.

These are guidelines for individual clinicians. Teams and departments can also help to reduce prescribing errors by reviewing their systems. Examples of actions include:

- Limiting formularies. Complex formularies with unnecessary duplication and confusing choices will increase the risk of prescribing or dispensing errors.
- Pharmacists attending ward rounds to review prescribing and check for drug interactions.
- Monitoring of drug charts on a systematic basis by pharmacy staff.
- Making sure there is easy access to drug information, either in paper or electronic form, on the wards and in clinics.
- Clear labelling of high risk drugs with good communication between staff.
- Computerized prescribing aids can help to check doses and interactions and alert clinical staff to possible dangers.

CLINICAL AUDIT

Clinical audit is a well-established method of reviewing clinical practice against agreed standards with the aim of identifying areas for improvement in quality of care. It has been defined as 'the systematic, critical analysis of the quality of clinical care, including the procedures used for diagnosis and treatment, the use of resources and the resulting outcome and quality of life of the patient. Simply put, it involves looking at what you or your colleagues are doing, learning from it and changing your practice. If we do not examine or review what we are doing in clinical practice, then we will never pick up our mistakes. This review must be structured and systematic if it is going to be accurate and believable.

There are six key steps in undertaking clinical audits (see Figure 6.4):

1. Choose your topic
2. Define standards
3. Collect data on past or current performance
4. Analyse and present these data to your colleagues
5. Identify areas of poor performance and implement change
6. Re-audit performance in the light of change.

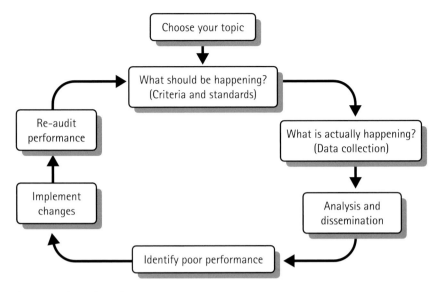

Fig 6.4 The audit cycle.

Remember that audit works best in improving care when it provides clinicians *with accurate and regular feedback on their own individual performance, compared to their peers*. While electronic patient records will allow such feedback at a click of a button in the future, at present such audits require time-consuming tracking of medical records and subsequent data extraction and analysis. So it is worth identifying a small number of important topics for regular, accurate audit and feedback rather than dozens of small, one-off audits that will have limited impact.

Choosing a topic

Most areas of clinical practice have well-established experience with clinical audit. Many professional bodies, such as the Royal Colleges, have set up and coordinated national audits for their specialist members. Before embarking on a new audit, always make sure you review the literature and talk to colleagues to find out what has been done locally and nationally on the topic.

If the audit is to lead to change, then it is essential that all your colleagues are aware and on board. Changing your own practice in the light of audit results can be relatively simple. The hard part comes with trying to change others, and ownership from the start is a vital part of this change process. Make sure that everyone agrees that the audit is important and will collaborate in it. This may involve different disciplines and primary and secondary care clinicians.

The audit topic should be centred around quality of patient care, and not on some quasi-research exercise for testing hypotheses. It should also be based on a topic for which there is clear evidence about what good care involves. If there is no good evidence then it will be difficult to agree what standards of care should be.

Box 6.7   Checklist for choosing a topic for audit

1. Is the topic an important public health problem in terms of size (prevalence or incidence), cost to the health service or clinical risk to patients?
2. Is there evidence that current quality of patient care should be improved?
3. Is this change in patient care achievable?
4. Are there measurable clinical outcomes which can be used to monitor change?
5. Is there good research evidence available about the most clinically effective and cost-effective management of patients?
6. Does the audit have a clear patient focus?
7. Is there multidisciplinary involvement?
8. Is there inter-sectoral involvement between primary and secondary care?
9. Are there links to education and professional development to implement change?

Box 6.7 provides a checklist for choosing audit topics. This should provide a reference for deciding on the benefits and feasibility of audits.

Defining standards

Before evaluating clinical performance you need to define what good practice actually involves. By defining standards of good care you can then determine how local care measures up against them. Defining standards also helps to clarify what exactly you want to measure.

Quality standards are often defined in terms of structure, process and outcome, and this can provide a useful framework for undertaking audit.

- Structure measures the physical environment of health care such as buildings, facilities, equipment, staff and case records. This can be described as what you need.
- Process describes the delivery of health care, or what you actually do. For example, prescribing, investigations, communication and clinical decision-making.
- Outcome describes the health status of the patient, or what you ultimately want to achieve. For example, reduced mortality, increased quality of life, reduced disability, lowered blood pressure.

The most important of these components for assessing quality of care is outcome. However, this is often the hardest to measure and we often tend to focus on process measures when auditing performance. Wherever possible a combination of both process and outcome measures should be used, and the process measures should be based on aspects of care that are important in achieving good outcomes.

So for example, an audit of patients admitted with acute myocardial infarction would measure an outcome of mortality, using national comparisons to define a standard (10% mortality). It would collate process measures such as the proportion of patients who received thrombolysis (and the pain to needle time), aspirin and beta blockers, as these are all components of clinical care that are well established as effective in improving outcomes. Standards should be set from those in the literature; for example, taking into consideration contra-indications, 80% of patients should receive thrombolysis and 90% aspirin.

Collecting data

There are two main sources of data for audit. First, routine data are collected on every patient. This includes information such as age, sex, diagnosis, length of stay, operations and mortality. The main advantage of this information is that it is easily available on hospital or practice information systems and can provide a useful starting point to describe patient characteristics and activity. However, it is very limited in what it tells us about quality of care and is frequently inaccurate.

The second and more valuable source of data is the patient records. These contain all the important details on the process and outcome of health care. Case note review can be used to examine the care of a large number of patients, or just one or two patients in whom there were significant events (death or complications).

A number of steps must be taken before you launch into data collection.

1. Define what information you need to record from each patient record. There is a common tendency to want to record too much detail, most of which will turn out to be useless. The level of detail must be balanced by the effort involved in extracting and analysing all the information. Common variables will include patient details (age, sex); diagnosis; co-morbidity; interventions; complications.
2. Design and pilot a data extraction sheet. This should be easy to complete, code and analyse. Piloting is a key part of any audit as it helps avoid crucial mistakes such as collecting the wrong information or missing out important information. Piloting also helps to assess the feasibility of the audit and make adaptations to ensure that it is successful.
3. Select your sample. Most clinicians know that research must be rigorously conducted and bias avoided if the results are to be believed. For some reason, when it comes to audit, many consider that any old methodology will suffice. Biased audit will not provide valid results and so will be wasted effort. The two main forms of sampling are:

   (i) Comprehensive: every patient record over a stated time period is reviewed. This is possible if there are limited numbers with the condition of interest, or if there are resources available.
   (ii) Random: use random number tables (in statistical books or on computer spreadsheets) in conjunction with a list of your patients to obtain a random sample. This will provide a bias-free sample. An alternative is to undertake systematic sampling of every 5th/10th patient from your list.

Every effort should then be made to track down all the requested records. The records that are difficult to obtain (e.g. because the patient has died or is under ongoing care because of complications) may be the records that contain the most valuable information.

Sample size is not as important an issue as it is in clinical trials where statistical power must be demonstrated. It is often governed by resources available. However, you should estimate a sample size that will be sufficient to provide generalizable and valid results.

A common finding from retrospective case note audit is that there are large gaps in the information recorded and it is impossible to collate the required audit data. This reflects the limitations of relying on retrospective record review. For important clinical topics (e.g. cancer care or myocardial infarction) *prospective* data collection should be considered. This allows greater completeness and accuracy of information recording. With computerized records, this will become increasingly the norm; however, in the meantime, specific databases for such audits have to be maintained. Some of the many examples of these include ICNARC for intensive care patients, and NAOMI for myocardial infarction. Box 6.8 shows an example of a prospective audit.

Box 6.8   Audit example: oxygen prescribing on respiratory wards

Topic: Oxygen treatment is common in hospital and may be lethal if inadequately prescribed.

Standards: A review of the medical literature provided standards for safe and effective delivery of oxygen.

Data collection: Details about oxygen prescribing were collected from patient records prospectively for all patients in two respiratory wards over a 2-month period.

Analysis: 86 patients were identified. Prescriptions were absent or inaccurate for 82% of patients.

Review and feedback: Discussion of the results revealed the lack of knowledge that junior doctors had about safe and effective oxygen prescribing. A prescription chart for oxygen was developed to help guide prescribing of type of delivery device, concentration and flow rate.

Re-audit: Following introduction of the oxygen prescription chart the audit was repeated. 92 patients were identified in the second audit. Only 22% of patients had absent or inaccurate prescriptions.

Analysing information

Data protection is an issue of great public concern, so care must be taken to ensure that confidentiality and security of patient information are paramount.

With small audits it may be possible to go through the results and summarize them manually. However, for most audits, the large amount of information collected and analysed makes this laborious. Greater flexibility and efficiency will be gained from using a computer spreadsheet or database. Each recorded item should be coded (for example, sex: female = 1, male = 2; or postoperative complications: wound infection = 1, deep venous thrombosis = 2, pulmonary embolism = 3, etc.). This coded information can then be analysed and summarized.

There are commercial systems that can be used for scanning data sheets in and collating results. These include Formic and Teleform. An example for use in a prospective audit of cataract surgery is shown in Figure 6.5.

Most analysis of audit data will be descriptive. This will provide summary statistics of frequencies, means, modes, standard deviations and temporal trends. Where databases are sufficiently large then correlation and

ONE PAGE CATARACT AUDIT – EYE SPECIFIC

As this page is going to be scanned it is important to complete the form correctly. Please print carefully inside the boxes and mark tick-box choices with a cross like so ☒ Thanks.

Please stick Patient ID Label here without obscuring the black locator block above

FINAL DRAFT

VA codes				
01 = 6/6 or better	04 = 6/18	07 = 6/60	10 = CF,HM	99 = unknown
02 = 6/9	05 = 6/24	08 = 3/60	11 = PL	
03 = 6/12	06 = 6/36	09 = 1/60	12 = NPL	

Q1 Consultant List ☐ A ☐ B ☐ C ☐ D ☐ E ☐ F

Q2 Grade of Surgeon ☐ Consultant ☐ Snr Reg./Registrar ☐ SHO ☐ Other

Q3 Operation ☐ Right eye ☐ Left eye **Q4** Type of Operation ☐ Phaco ☐ ECCE

Q5 Operation eye ☐ First ☐ Second **Q6** Visual acuity – Best corrected (with glasses, CL or pin hole) – At Pre-assessment in eye

Q7 Anaesthetic ☐ L.A. ☐ G.A. due for operation ☐☐

Q8 Comorbidity – Before Surgery – Operated eye

☐ None

☐ Diabetic retinopathy (background maculopathy, preproliferative, proliferative)

☐ ARMD (drusen, RPE changes, geographic atrophy neovascularization, haemorrhage, disciform scar)

☐ Amblyopia

☐ Glaucoma   Other – please specify

Q9 Date surgery performed

D D   M M   Y Y Y Y
☐☐ ☐☐ ☐☐☐☐

Q10 Visual acuity – Best corrected (with glasses, CL or pin hole) – At final refraction in operated eye
☐☐

Q11 Complications in eye that had cataract surgery

☐ None
☐ Sustained raised IOP
☐ External eye infection
☐ Vitreous to section
☐ Persistent corneal oedema
☐ Persistent severe uveitis
☐ Iris abnormality
☐ Posterior capsule opacity
☐ Posterior capsular tear

☐ Cystoid macular oedema
☐ Retinal tear
☐ Retinal detachment
☐ Had to convert to ECCE
☐ Refractive surprise/unintended anisometropia
☐ Endophthalmitis

Other, please specify below

Q12 If the patient's visual activity in operated eye is worse than 6/12 at final refraction then can it be attributed to pre-existing comorbidity?

☐ Yes   ☐ No   ☐ Not applicable

Fig. 6.5 Data recording sheet for automatic scanning.

significance testing may be useful. Seek help if you are uncertain about what statistical testing to perform and how to carry it out.

The next step is to present the information. Common mistakes in presenting audit results are either to list endless numbers and frequencies, or to go over the top and prepare all-singing, three-dimensional graphs summarizing just a small amount of information. Histograms, bar charts, pie charts and time trend graphs will be sufficient for most presentations. Good, clear presentation is as important as good data collection, but keep it simple and concentrate on the lessons rather than the details. Lastly, make sure that confidentiality is maintained and any feedback to the group is anonymized if the results are sensitive.

Review performance and implement change

The presentation of results will identify standards of care that are not being met and provide objective evidence about clinical performance to balance subjective opinions. It will also demonstrate what standards are being met and examples of good practice. These successes should be highlighted just as much as the failures to allow everybody a collective pat on the back.

Feedback of clinical performance can be a powerful force for promoting change where there is complacency about individual and departmental practice. The feedback should be to the whole department or clinical governance group so that open discussion can take place about the results and there can be an honest appraisal of why good or poor performance occurred. Ensure that everybody has the opportunity to attend and participate. Try and involve people by making the session as interactive as possible, not just the same old voices monopolizing the discussion.

The next step is to agree on what action is needed to improve performance. If the review of the audit produces debate but no action then it is wasted. Individuals may change their practice, but clinical performance relies on teamwork and team changes. Changing practice is not easy (see Chapter 7). It requires time, resources and ownership from the different members of the department or group. Make sure that everybody is signed up to the changes and don't be afraid to allocate various roles and responsibilities to different individuals so that everyone is clear about what they have to do, and by when. Vagueness is the kiss of death to adopting and implementing change.

Action taken to improve performance may involve setting up a training session for staff, an induction workshop for new doctors, clinical guidelines, changes to the process of care such as how and where patients are admitted, or documentation in records.

Re-audit

Like puppies, audit should be for life, not just for Christmas. Audit is an ongoing cycle and re-audit is the next rotation. This allows change and progress (and hopefully improvement) to be demonstrated after changes

---

Box 6.9   Audit example: thromboprophylaxis in surgery

Topic: Thromboembolism is a common cause of postoperative morbidity and mortality which can be prevented by using appropriate prophylactic measures.

Standards: Standards were defined from national guidelines from the Royal College of Surgeons.

Data collection: Details were collected for all surgical inpatients regarding thromboprophylaxis received and patient risk factors for a 3-month period.

Analysis: 170 patients were included in the audit. Only 47% had received appropriate thromboprophylaxis according to their risk assessment.

Review and feedback: Subsequent discussion in the surgical clinical governance meeting acknowledged substandard care. Local guidelines were developed for use on the wards. A formal risk assessment form was introduced for both nursing and medical staff to score the risk for patients. A number of educational events were held for staff about the guidelines and scoring system.

Re-audit: 165 patients were included in the 2-month follow-up audit. The number of patients who had received appropriate thromboprophylaxis had increased to 78%.

---

have been put into practice to reduce poor performance. It also reinforces lessons and encourages sustainability of change. Old habits die hard and it is common for such old practice habits to creep back into the routine. Re-audit allows a review of performance over time.

As mentioned above, the best form of audit is one that involves prospective data collection, and if the topic is important enough to justify the resources required to allow this, then such a system should be considered.

NATIONAL CONFIDENTIAL ENQUIRIES

There are four national Confidential Enquiries that come under the umbrella of the National Institute of Clinical Excellence. These collate information on deaths in four key areas and feed this information back to hospitals and health professionals on an anonymized basis. This allows a systematic and critical examination of all deaths to take place by peer-review groups who then provide a summary of lessons to be learnt and recommendations for future practice. These deaths are often rare events and so individual clinicians are unable to learn these valuable lessons from their own limited experience.

Simply participating and submitting information to these enquiries may improve quality of care by promoting greater awareness and reflection in participating clinicians. However, simply feeding back the lessons of each enquiry to individual clinicians will not necessarily lead to change. When annual reports are disseminated by these enquiries they should be reviewed by relevant clinical teams in their clinical governance framework. Recommendations should be discussed and action agreed, implemented and audited.

Confidential Enquiry into Stillbirths and Deaths in Infancy (CESDI)

This was established in 1992 to improve the understanding of how the risks of death in late fetal life (20 weeks) up to infancy (1 year) might be reduced. It aims to identify and highlight risks which can be attributed to suboptimal clinical care. Some deaths, for example cot deaths, are rare and so this national reporting system allows lessons to be learnt that would otherwise have been missed.

Data on some 10 000 deaths annually are notified to a network of regional coordinators in England, Wales and Northern Ireland. These are collated by CESDI and then external multidisciplinary enquiry panels examine particular subsets of mortality (e.g. prematurity, intrapartum deaths > 2.5 kg) with the aim of identifying weaknesses in systems of care and advising on how improvements can be made.

Recent examples of areas covered by CESDI include breech presentation, obstetric anaesthetic complications and delays, sudden unexpected deaths in infancy.

National Confidential Enquiry into Perioperative Deaths (NCEPOD)

This independent body was established in 1987. Its aim is to review clinical practice and identify potentially remediable factors in the practice of anaesthesia, surgery and other invasive medical procedures. In 2002 it extended this review to include all deaths of patients admitted under medical care and/or within 30 days of gastrointestinal endoscopy.

Details are collected on all deaths that occur in hospital within 30 days of a surgical procedure by local NCEPOD coordinators. These are then sent to the national office for collation and analysis. A sample of the reported deaths (e.g. 10% of cases) is randomly selected for detailed review to examine the quality of health care delivery. Recommendations from the analysis and review of collected data are made in annual reports.

Recent examples of areas highlighted include inadequacies of intensive care facilities, poor documentation, poor teamwork and communication, problems with minimally invasive surgery, failures in care of children and the elderly, lack of adequate involvement of senior staff in decision-making, knowing when not to operate on very sick patients. Box 6.10 summarizes findings from the NCEPOD report.

Confidential Enquiry into Maternal Deaths

This is the longest running confidential enquiry, having been established in 1952. Maternal deaths are rare in developed countries. This hinders individuals from learning lessons about how such deaths can be avoided. By collation and analysis of all deaths nationally, general lessons can be drawn.

Between 1994 and 1996 there were 376 deaths, some of which were unavoidable, but some of which could have been prevented through improved standards of health care delivery.

Examples of substandard care include failure to detect problems in pregnancy such as ectopic pregnancies, pre-eclampsia, pulmonary emboli; failure of senior staff in attending cases or delegating decisions; lack of teamwork; lack of departmental guidelines.

Confidential Inquiry into Suicides and Homicides by People with Mental Illness

This inquiry investigates anonymized information from a sample of people who have committed suicide (about 1200 per year) after being in contact with mental health services during the previous 12 months. It also investigates homicides involving people who have been in contact with mental health services at any time (about 40 per year).

These confidential enquiries have two main weaknesses. First, participation is voluntary and so some deaths are not included. For NCEPOD the participation rate is about 80%. Higher coverage for the Confidential Inquiry into Suicides and Homicides is achieved by using other sources of information in addition to reporting.

Box 6.10   2001 NCEPOD Report findings

Anaesthesia and surgery
- Some hospitals deny certain patients access to HDUs
- Central venous pressure monitoring was used in 44% of patients, but another 13% would have benefited from it

General anaesthesia with regional analgesia
- Regional analgesia combined with general anaesthesia may precipitate hypotension, especially in those who are septic or dehydrated
- Anaesthetists should be cautious about the dose of local anaesthetic used on patients predisposed to hypotension

Aortic stenosis
- Whenever possible, anaesthetists should get a preoperative echocardiogram of the aortic valve
- Echocardiography services should be better funded

Perioperative care
- Timing of operations was often 'inappropriate' to the patient's state
- CVP lines were 'poorly managed' on the wards

Surgery in general
- Fluid balance and incontinence to be 'proactively managed'

Vascular surgery
- Correction of coagulopathy is important in the management of bleeding in surgery for ruptured abdominal aortic aneurysms
- MRSA infection is a hazard for surgical patients

Histology
- A third of histology reports contained insufficient information to support tumour staging and clinical management

---

Second, although each will make regular recommendations based on their review of cases, there is no compulsion to follow these recommendations, and no method of monitoring implementation of the recommendations. A review of the confidential enquiries is currently underway in the NHS and changes about confidentiality may well take place.

Local action

Reporting deaths for the confidential enquiries should be a straightforward process. However, in reality it can be a time-consuming exercise of form-filling and note-chasing. Case notes are often lost in the dark depths of coroners' offices, or lie guiltily in the corner of a secretary's room, waiting for reports.

Deaths reflect one extreme outcome of clinical care, and may not provide lessons for improvement. Examining morbidity or critical incidents where death was avoided will often be more informative and constructive. However, deaths are easy to measure, and will inevitably continue to be the focus of national audits.

Enquiry reports from a hospital should be regularly audited and reviewed. The foundation for this should include the following:

- Identified senior clinician from each speciality responsible for coordinating the audit in the hospital.
- Identified clinical governance support facilitator to receive case notes of all relevant patient deaths and ensure that appropriate clinicians complete the report forms to agreed timescales.
- Regular audit and case studies of local deaths. This should be directed by the local coordinator, but the audit or case note review should be undertaken by a clinical team unconnected to the care being assessed. As with the national enquiries, different themes can be chosen for specific audits, such as deaths out-of-hours, or deaths in the elderly. Audit of the case notes should record standards of the different aspects of care such as preoperative preparation and postoperative fluid replacement.
- Regular quarterly or biannual review meetings to discuss local and national results. This should be multidisciplinary and include all relevant clinical specialities. Deaths are rarely 'surgical' deaths, 'anaesthetic' deaths or 'orthopaedic' deaths – there will be many different causes from different steps in the patient pathway.
- Regular review of local results by the hospital clinical governance committee. Such senior review is essential for achieving objectivity and promoting action on results.

STATISTICAL PROCESS CONTROL AND THE USE OF CONTROL CHARTS

One of the triggers for the introduction of clinical governance was the recognition of wide variations in standards of care (e.g. treatment rates or death rates) in the NHS. Such variation is so often described as 'unacceptable' that the two words have become natural partners. However, variation in outcomes is a natural result of all complex processes and health care is no exception. If we are to make genuine improvements in the quality of health care then we must recognize variations in outcomes, understand their causes and identify problems. Averages in performance measures have traditionally been used to monitor quality. However, averages by their nature will conceal variation and because they are calculated from retrospective data, will never be timely enough to lead to quick changes.

One method of monitoring and reviewing measurements of quality of care is by using statistical process control charts.[1,2] Control charts have been in common use for monitoring and improving quality in many industries and have recently been adopted in health care settings. Outcome data are plotted over time (or may compare different 'units' such as general practices or hospitals). The mean is plotted and limits are calculated for three **sigmas** (equivalent to 99.8% confidence intervals) above and below the mean. Outcomes at times (or in units) beyond these limits may be considered special and an assignable cause for the variation may be sought. Time points (or units) within the limits should be considered to be the same, as no assignable cause can be found to account for the variation between time points (or units).

The statistical methods used in control charts are very robust. The presentation of the control charts is simple and can be understood by most health professionals. Rather than providing snapshots of information like other forms of data presentation and charts, it allows data to be presented continuously over time. Such data can be individual patient data (e.g. INRs of a patient on anticoagulation therapy) or aggregated patient data (e.g. waiting times for an outpatient clinic or inpatient infection rates).

Control charts also provide a useful method of monitoring variation in performance between hospitals. Traditional league tables of performance indicators such as mortality rates tend to unfairly stigmatize those hospitals at the bottom of the league when factors such as case mix or chance variation may be responsible. Control charts can monitor performance without ranking and with clearer differentiation between random variation and special causes.

Figure 6.6 shows the percentage of cervical cytology smear tests rejected as inadequate in a pathology laboratory. It provides an easily interpretable chart showing average performance, upper and lower control limits (in this context this is 3 sigma from the mean,) and up-to-date quarterly data which can be compared to past performance, so that previous data are not forgotten.

The chart shows a rise in inadequate smear tests to about 12% which prompted a review of local practices. This review revealed recent changes in processing of smear tests and a high number of abnormal smears being sent by trainer general practitioners and practice nurses. Changes were made as to how smears were read and a training session was held for those taking smear tests. The control chart allowed improvements to be monitored. Not only was the 'special cause' variation reduced, but also the wider training programme allowed 'common cause' variation to be 'reset' at a lower mean level.

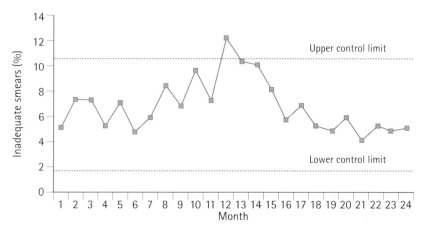

Fig. 6.6   Control chart of inadequate cervical smears.

REFERENCES

1. Mohammed AM, Cheng KK, Rouse A, Marshall T. Bristol, Shipman, and clinical governance: Shewhart's forgotten lessons. *Lancet* 2001; **357**: 463–467.
2. Adab P, Rouse AM, Mohammed AM, Marshall T. Performance league tables: the NHS deserves better. *BMJ* 2002; **324**: 95–98).

Clinical guidelines and changing clinical practice

7

This chapter concentrates on clinical guidelines. It covers the following areas:

- Rationale for guidelines
- How to develop guidelines
- Changing clinical practice: implementing guidelines
- Examples of implementation programmes
- Care pathways.

What happens when audits, critical incident reviews or feedback of complaints or clinical risk reports demonstrate gaps in the quality of care? The next step after these reviews of performance is to try to get colleagues on a ward, in a hospital or across a district to improve their clinical practice in line with the recommended standards. One of the most common suggestions for doing this is 'let's write a guideline'. Someone (usually a junior doctor or the local expert) then goes off, sits down at their kitchen table that night and writes what they think should be best practice. This is typed up and circulated to all interested parties who either (a) consign it to the rubbish bin with that day's excess of post or (b) file it for future reference in a soon forgotten location. Practice then carries on as before and no one should be too surprised when a repeat review of performance shows no change.

In recent years there has been an enormous expansion in the development and dissemination of guidelines. It has become an industry itself with drug companies and academic or professional institutions competing with each other to churn out the greatest number. If you go to most wards or doctors' offices you will find dusty tomes of clinical guidelines, sometimes occupying entire shelves, and yet most lie unread and unused. So why bother with guidelines? Just as with most medicines, it is not simply a question of ingredients and dispensing; it is more important how they are used in practice.

This chapter will discuss the potential benefits of clinical guidelines, how to develop them and how to get colleagues to use them.

WHAT ARE GUIDELINES AND DO THEY WORK?

Guidelines have been defined by the Institute of Medicine as 'systematically developed statements which assist clinicians and patients in making decisions about appropriate treatment for specific conditions'. Other terms have been used to describe guidelines, such as protocols or algorithms, but guidelines are the preferred description. It could be argued that many clinical textbooks are just overgrown guidelines, but clinical guidelines tend to imply summaries of the knowledge to use as quick references in clinical practice.

Recent interest in guidelines has been motivated by a number of reasons:

- Widespread variation in practice. If you examine rates of operating, prescribing or use of diagnostic tests then you find large variations, not just between different areas in the country but also between different hospitals in the same district and different clinicians in the same department. We all know of the usual problem of having to check which consultant the patient is under because Dr Smith prefers this treatment, whereas Dr Brown prefers the opposite. While there are many areas of uncertainty in medicine, most observers agree that wide variation is not acceptable for a national health service. Guidelines offer the potential to describe best practice for all to follow.
- Long delays in the uptake of evidence. It took over 100 years for the finding that limes prevented scurvy to be put into practice in the British navies. Such delays in the introduction of effective treatments may be shorter these days, but if you look at common clinical topics such as asthma, hypertension or *Helicobacter pylori* eradication you can show delays of 10 and 20 years. Guidelines offer the potential to reduce these delays by providing up-to-date evidence for clinicians.
- Summaries of the evidence. Medical knowledge is complex and ever changing. It can be confusing to those outside a particular clinical specialism trying to get to grips with the conflicting aspects of the latest research studies. Most professionals do not have the time to acquire in-depth understanding of the large number of medical fields, and rather than have to consult wordy textbooks, they would prefer to have summaries of the evidence to help make decisions in their day-to-day lives.
- Encourage explicit decision-making. Much of our clinical decision-making is jumbled and implicit. If a patient asks us why we have decided on a particular option or treatment, we tend to be defensive and paternal. Inside our heads lie hundreds of thousands of bits of information from teachings, books, journals, experience and anecdote. How we use all this information often tends to be inconsistent and dependent on our most recent influences. Guidelines offer a structure for our decision-making, and because they are written down, they can be used by patients themselves to inform choices.

Guidelines can offer a good opportunity for team-building and inter-professional collaboration. They also provide standards for audit. However, the most important reason for using guidelines would be if they improve patient care. But do they? As with any other health care intervention, the evidence of effectiveness of guidelines should be systematically reviewed.

A large number of rigorous clinical trials have been undertaken to evaluate the effect of clinical guidelines. A Cochrane systematic review of these trials has shown that clinical guidelines do significantly improve both the process and more importantly the outcome of patient care. However, for guidelines to be effective they need to be 1) scientifically valid and 2) appropriately developed, disseminated and implemented.

HOW TO DEVELOP A GUIDELINE

Nearly all health professionals will have reason to use clinical guidelines. Many will want to develop specific guidelines for use in their hospital or practice. This section describes how to develop an effective guideline (Figure 7.1).

Step 1: Choose the topic

1. *Is it important?* There is little point spending precious time and effort on a guideline for viral haemorrhagic fever if your hospital treats one case every 5 years. One of the potential problems with clinical guidelines is that they tend to multiply. It is better to develop guidelines for a few, important clinical conditions that will be used than hundreds of guidelines for every conceivable topic that end up causing confusion. Large numbers of guidelines soon develop into a textbook that collects dust on a shelf.

   The usual criterion for choosing a guideline topic is that it should have an important health impact in terms of either:

   - numbers of patients, e.g. asthma or angina
   - risk to life or health, e.g. acute meningitis or gastrointestinal haemorrhage
   - cost to the health service, e.g. expensive drugs for use in multiple sclerosis or ovarian cancer.

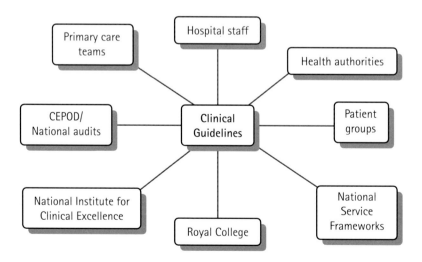

Fig. 7.1 Stakeholders for initiating and developing clinical guidelines.

The guideline can cover aspects of clinical care such as how to manage a patient with chest pain or epilepsy; diagnosis and investigation, such as investigation of deep venous thrombosis of the calf; or prescribing, such as antibiotic use.

2. *Is there room for improvement*? If an audit shows that everyone is following best practice then there is little point in putting a lot of work into reiterating this. If, however, there is evidence of variation in practice, inappropriate use of investigations or treatments, or critical incidents that have caused concern, then guidelines may be of value.

3. *Is there an evidence-base*? If there is variation because no one agrees what the evidence is then there may be brick walls ahead. Avoid uncertainty and controversy and stick to guidelines for which you are likely to obtain consensus.

Step 2: Identify barriers and incentives

Spending a bit of time at the start of a new topic in seeking to understand potential barriers and incentives to change as well as local politics is essential if success is to be achieved. Potential barriers may include:

- Lack of time. There is never enough time, but improving patient care must be a priority, and good guidelines may save time in the end by reducing inappropriate referrals or complications.
- Lack of funding. Insufficient local services, e.g. low numbers of staff or diagnostic services may hinder change. Involvement of managers may be important.
- Organizational factors. Lack of support from the hospital or different priorities.
- Professional factors. Conflict between different demands from different disciplines or between professional and patient needs.
- Individual factors. Lack of knowledge or skills in local staff.

Try to link guidelines with incentives such as resource allocation, feedback of performance or training. Subsequent motivation for change may be greater.

Discuss the topic with key clinicians and other staff in the district. Ask them to identify the barriers and incentives, and find out how they would set about the task of developing guidelines or improving practice. Find out what current practice is and why it differs from best practice. Assess whether local consensus is achievable and whether subsequent change is likely.

Step 3: Choose the group

Guideline development has moved on from being a solitary affair with a kitchen table. Involving the right people in development is important for two reasons. Firstly, the care of a patient depends on different health professionals. Each different professional group will have their own important contributions to make to a guideline and useful messages to get across. Secondly, if the guideline is to be effective then different professionals must be signed up to it. If one group has been left out then they are unlikely to feel particularly motivated to adhere to the guidelines developed. The right membership will promote the right credibility and it is important to start by thinking who the guideline is aimed at (Box 7.1).

Crossing the interface between primary and secondary care is often neglected when it comes to guidelines. There is a tendency to have one rule for hospital care and one for the rest. While many of the patients seen in hospital will be different from those seen in primary care (in severity of illness for instance), the evidence base for treatment or investigation will be substantially the same. So, for example, upper gastrointestinal endoscopy for a patient in hospital should not be governed by different guidance just because it is easy to access.

Few patients are aware of the artificial distinction between primary and secondary care. Each contact is just another stop on their health journey. Clinical guidelines need to acknowledge this movement across 'borders'.

The other frequently forgotten group for involvement in guideline development is the managers. This is short-sighted as there will be little sympathy if you turn up 6 months after the guidelines have been agreed saying you need a new drug, or more staff or another echo machine. Managers will have control of staff and resources, and they are better on-side than off-field.

One last, but very important, group is the patients themselves. In many cases this may not be appropriate, for example, in acute emergency guidelines or diagnostics. However, more and more patients want to know the basis of clinical decision-making, particularly in chronic diseases such as diabetes, epilepsy or angina. Where possible a patient should be included in the group, or carers (e.g. in the case of stroke patients). Ask around and select someone who will be assertive enough to contribute in a potentially intimidating professional environment.

Box 7.1   Choosing a guideline development group

Leadership: does the group have a chair who has the skills of communication and facilitation to develop consensus guidelines?

Expertise: are the staff with the specialist knowledge on hand?

Medical staff: are the different specialties represented? If the guideline is aimed at junior doctors, are they represented?

Nursing and therapy staff: few topics are the sole preserve of doctors and most other health professionals will have knowledge and know-how about particular topics.

Primary care: again, few topics are the sole preserve of hospital care, and local general practitioners and practice nurses should be invited if the guidelines will impact on them.

Managers: many guidelines have implications of costs or changes in demand for particular services.

Administrative or project management support: clinical governance departments should ensure that they have staff with the skills to support the process.

Patients: This may be difficult, and not always appropriate, but guidelines are all about improving patient care, and their voice should be heard.

Clinical guidelines and changing clinical practice

Guideline discussions are often very technical and the environment can be intimidating. Alternative methods of obtaining patient involvement should be considered, such as running separate focus groups to allow the consensus group to be informed by what patients and their carers think are the important points for inclusion in guidelines.

Step 4: Set the agenda

Once you have everybody in the same room you need to ensure that they all understand why they are there and what they need to do. Start by making sure that everyone knows who each member is and why they are there, and check that no one is missing. Addressing the following questions will help you and the group:

1. What is the aim of the group? This is usually to develop valid and evidence-based guidelines for a particular clinical area.
2. What is the remit? How broad is the clinical area? If the guidelines are for the management of patients with stroke, will they cover acute, diagnostic or rehabilitation aspects?
3. How long will it take? Time is precious, and although much can be achieved outside meetings, the group has to agree to the commitment involved. Estimate the time it will take to develop and then implement the guidelines.

Step 5: Identify valid guidelines

For a guideline to be valid it should be based on a systematic review of the available research evidence on the particular clinical topic (see Chapter 4). Just as traditional reviews of the evidence can be haphazard and biased, so can clinical guidelines. Guideline reviewers should use explicit standards for appraising and synthesizing this research evidence, otherwise there is the danger that guideline recommendations will be inaccurate or biased because of omissions in relevant evidence or because of the particular beliefs or prejudices of the guideline developers. An example of evidence grading for guideline recommendations is given in Box 7.2.

Unfortunately, such systematic guideline development can be very time-consuming and may require particular skills. Local guideline groups are rarely equipped for such undertakings, and indeed should not be encouraged to try – it is not necessarily a wise use of local staff time and resources. Guidelines have been developed in most clinical areas and the starting point for most local guideline development should be a search for national or other local guidelines.

Box 7.2　Grading the evidence for guideline recommendations

A – based on randomized controlled trials or systematic reviews
B – based on robust experimental or observational studies
C – based on national expert consensus opinion
D – based on local expert consensus opinion

Box 7.3   Checklist for assessing the validity of clinical guidelines

1. Clear indication of the aim of the guidelines, the target patient population and the clinical setting for their use
2. Clear indication as to who developed the guidelines and how they were funded
3. Appropriate representation of different disciplines on the development group
4. Clear methodology as to how the evidence was searched and appraised
5. Description of how recommendations were made by the guideline development group
6. Grading of evidence to support recommendations
7. Indication of review date when guidelines should be updated
8. Consideration of cost-effectiveness as well as clinical effectiveness of recommendations

---

Start by searching library databases such as Medline. Check with the National Institute for Clinical Excellence as to whether there are national guidelines or plans for covering the topic. Try the professional organizations such as the Royal Colleges. Use local networks to find out what work has been done elsewhere. Then collate all the guidelines you find.

The next step is to appraise the guidelines to determine which are the most valid. This can often be difficult as few guidelines give details about how they were developed or the basis for the recommendations. There are tools for appraising guidelines, such as the St George's guideline appraisal instrument, although these can be too detailed. Box 7.3 provides a basic checklist for assessing the validity of a guideline. The guideline should be clear about the patient population and clinical context it covers. Recommendations should be supported by explicit strength of evidence. Methodology should be described and a review date given.

Step 6: Obtain consensus

Guidelines and supporting evidence should be circulated to the group. In a perfect world you could identify suitably valid guidelines, approve them with a large group rubber stamp and stick them on the shelf on the ward or in the clinic. Simple endorsement may sometimes be all that is needed, but clinical practice can be hard to change and the process of change is important. Your consensus group needs to meet and discuss the guidelines. This ensures that all the stakeholders are signed up to the recommendations and provides an excellent opportunity to spend some protected time reflecting on what current practice is and what it should be.

It is always interesting to review guidelines and their recommendations in a group. It reveals different practices between different clinicians – different drugs or doses used, different use of investigations, different surgical techniques. It allows debate about what is best practice, backed up by explicit levels of evidence. It provides a forum for different voices that may have previously been ignored. It also identifies the potential barriers to adopting local guidelines; for example, lack of diagnostic equipment such as echocardiography to diagnose heart failure, restricted access because of waiting times that limit the diagnosis of epilepsy or disagreement with the evidence such as grommet insertions for glue ear.

Using the circulated guidelines and evidence as a foundation, adaptations can be made to local circumstances. The group should take into account the specific health needs of the local population and the availability of current services. Changes agreed by the group can be made and circulated outside the meeting or discussed at a subsequent meeting. Circulate early drafts to people outside the group – the wider the net is cast in seeking people's opinion, the earlier disagreements can be resolved and ownership encouraged.

Step 7: Presentation and access

With consensus achieved the next step is to package the guidelines so that they will be accessible and readable. Many national guidelines, and some local guidelines, tend to end up as bulky tomes with slabs of text and reams of references. Guidelines should be quick reference documents for busy clinicians making frequent clinical decisions. So design and presentation are important. Having invested so much effort in developing the guidelines, it is worth spending a bit of time to make sure they are used.

There is no single method for presentation of guidelines. Some may be best conveyed as algorithms or flow charts, with the diagnosis as the starting point (e.g. endometrial carcinoma). However, patients tend not to be aware of the

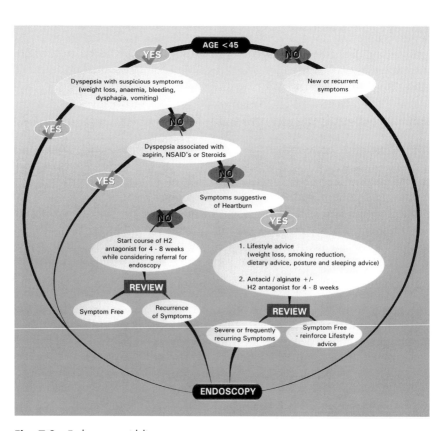

Fig. 7.2 Endoscopy guidelines.

Clinical guidelines and changing clinical practice

need to present with a diagnosis, and the symptom may be the most suitable starting point (e.g. post-menopausal bleeding).

Cheap and easy-to-use computer design packages are now widely available, and it is worth thinking about transferring dull lists of recommendations into more eye-catching formats (Figure 7.2).

Finally, try and ensure that the guidelines are accessible. Where are they going to be used most? Which staff are going to use them and where do they go for information? A few years ago there was an interesting little trial published which randomized two junior doctors' residences. In the intervention residence posters describing patient resuscitation methods were stuck on the back of toilet doors. The other residence acted as the control. After a few weeks the researchers assessed both groups of junior doctors and found that those allocated to the posters in the toilets had significantly greater knowledge about how to resuscitate patients.

The logical extreme of guideline posters could be to wallpaper wards and residences with them. This is obviously going too far, but there is no reason why important topics should not be promoted this way. Methods of dissemination to consider include:

- ward folders
- ward or clinic posters
- junior doctor handbooks
- desktop packs for clinics
- computers and even mouse-mats to improve access to the guidelines (Figure 7.3).

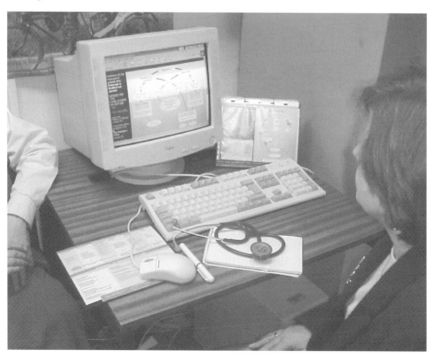

Fig. 7.3 Promotion of the use of guidelines via intranet/mouse-mats, etc.

Computer access either on stand-alone computers or on networks such as intranets will become increasingly important sources of guidelines (Box 7.4). This approach allows widespread access to guidelines throughout a hospital and between primary and secondary care. It also allows guidelines to be updated quickly and efficiently, without the danger of out-of-date guidelines lying around on wards being used by different staff.

All this work to develop one guideline may appear to be daunting. However, the outcome is not simply about a piece of paper with a flow chart on it. The outcome should be about better care of patients, a goal we all share and strive towards. This may involve time and effort, but along the way you will provide wonderful opportunities to:

- develop teamwork and communication
- reflect on current practices
- provide interactive and educational discussions about the evidence base behind clinical practice
- inspire different professionals towards a common goal
- set standards to measure future performance.

Be prepared for requests from the group for more!

Finally, time and resources are required to support this process and this should be identified clearly in departmental and organizational development plans. The process requires:

- leadership
- enthusiasm and energy
- careful planning and efficient use of time
- good communication with staff involved in the development and staff who will be using the guideline.

Box 7.4   Advantages of electronic publication

Ease of availability

Consistency of format

Guaranteed up to date and not out of date

Ease of alteration

Reminders when updating required

Ease of feedback comment

Can be used to develop newsgroup format about guideline

Guaranteed archiving

Ease of searching

Ease of adding references

Ease of notifying staff about new guidelines

Can be used to publish and archive newsletters, presentations, research details

Can be used to publish lessons learnt from clinical incidents

Allows copy to be placed easily in clinical record

CHANGING CLINICAL BEHAVIOUR: GETTING EVIDENCE INTO PRACTICE

So now you have a clinical guideline, based on the most up-to-date evidence and with the weight of local expertise behind it – what now? Sadly guidelines are not self-implementing and most clinicians recognize that they usually end up being added to the guideline mountain in the corner of the clinic room. All that effort of reviewing the evidence, obtaining consensus from all the different stakeholders and putting the information into a presentable form, and what happens next? They get posted out to all relevant professionals, printed in the relevant specialist journal and backed up by a few lectures from the authors.

This section will deal with how to change the clinical practice of your colleagues. There is pretty good evidence about what works in changing professional practice and implementation of guidelines (Box 7.5). There are no magic bullets for implementing change, but we do know that simply posting guidelines out, publishing them in journals and giving a few didactic lectures does not appear to have any clinical impact. So why are these methods the mainstay of professional development? Partly this may be due to habit, partly it may be due to lack of awareness about how ineffective these methods are.

The process of implementing guidelines and best practice is long and complex and dependent on many different patient, professional and contextual variables. Those who develop and promote clinical guidelines should not expect to step into a smooth and silent one-stop lift to reach their implementation heaven. Their journey is more by a cranky, old and dirty London

---

Box 7.5   Factors to promote uptake of guidelines

Qualities of guideline	– unbiased, authoritative, compatible with existing practices – clear, attractive format that is easy to understand – local or national priority – easily accessible
Implementation process	– combination of different approaches – practitioner-led – interactive and continually reinforced – ownership by relevant, professional groups
Characteristics of setting	– supportive national policy – clinical governance, National Service Frameworks – concern over litigation and accountability – effective local professional development and clinical networks, peer pressure – local opinion leaders and adequate resources – effective practice teams and organization
Characteristics of professional	– interest in clinical topic – good social and professional networks
Patient factors	– evidence underpinning guideline is generalizable to patients seen – patient preference and agreement

Underground escalator that lies broken for more time than it works (Figure 7.4 and Box 7.5). With the right spanners and lubricants they can improve their chances of reaching daylight.

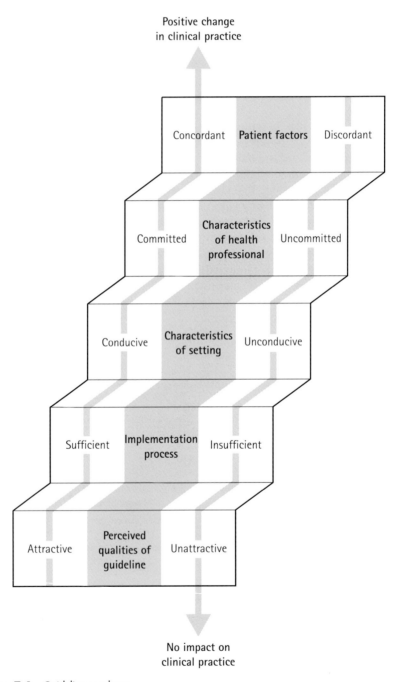

Fig. 7.4 Guideline escalator.

Clinical guidelines and changing clinical practice

Guideline developers should ensure that their product is well designed, and that the process of implementation is inclusive and sensitive to practice and organizational settings as well as the variable characteristics of the professionals and patients at whom the guideline is aimed. The process of implementation should be multi-faceted to target the various reasons for resistance to change and different learning needs. Different professionals have different ways of learning – some need only to read the guidelines to change. Some will need more intensive education, training and reminders. Others will need to learn new skills to adopt new practices.

Steps and interventions towards implementation

When you want to get your guideline, or any other clinical change, into routine practice there are a number of different approaches that can be followed. All require resources, some more than others. It would be great to copy the drug companies and send out academic detailers to every doctor, give out mugs with 'Prescribe Aspirin' on or set up snappy computer-aided prompts. However, this costs money. In practice we rely heavily on the use of existing resources.

The more effort that is put into the implementation phase, the more you will see change and subsequent improvements in patient care. The following steps and interventions should be considered:

1. *Contextual analysis.* Just as we need a diagnosis before we start treating a patient, so we need a contextual or diagnostic analysis before we start implementing change. Spend a bit of time at the start identifying the barriers and levers for change. Talk to relevant clinicians and managers to understand what will help and what will hinder implementation. Assess what the educational needs and objectives will be for the guideline implementation programme (see Chapter 5).
2. *Raise awareness.* Try to involve as many people as possible in commenting on the draft guidelines so that there is early ownership. Publicize the guidelines through local newsletters in the hospital or in primary care. Simple postal dissemination does not seem to be effective in promoting change; however, it may promote recognition and awareness that can then be built upon.
3. *Identify local 'opinion leaders'.* These are local health professionals who are considered to be influential in educating other staff about the guideline area. They are likely to be listened to and their clinical opinion is likely to be respected and adopted. They should be used to lead or support the educational and training events as part of the guideline implementation process. These opinion leaders usually have the enthusiasm to promote their messages, but may be limited by time constraints and some thought should go into how to use their time most efficiently.

   It is not always easy to identify clear opinion leaders in a particular field, but local knowledge and enquiry as part of the preliminary guideline work (see above) will usually provide suitable candidates. Characteristics of opinion leaders include: higher social status and ambition – greater knowledge and education, ability to show empathy and rationality, and higher public and professional profile.

4. Use *existing educational events* such as postgraduate lectures or clinical governance meetings (for hospital departments or primary care groups) to promote the guidelines to hospital staff and general practitioners.

   Didactic lectures are of dubious effectiveness, but are still the mainstay of medical education. Interactive and participatory sessions are more likely to promote change and subsequent guideline adoption. Involve your audience, listen to what they want to learn and provide concrete examples for them to learn from (Box 7.6).

5. *Educational outreach visits* by relevant medical and nursing specialists – taking the message out to the clinicians. These visits take place in the practice setting – for example, general practitioners' surgeries, or individual departments – and so tend to be more interactive and less formal. This is a strategy commonly used by the pharmaceutical industry and one that appears to be effective, yet it is one that the health service has been slow to adopt. The main reason for this inertia has been the lack of time and resources to send someone out to train other staff. However, it may be the only way to influence doctors who would not otherwise attend existing educational events. Such a targeted strategy may be valuable in changing the practice of those who deviate from guideline recommendations the most – a 10-minute discussion may prevent many time-consuming, inappropriate referrals.

6. *Prompts and reminders* can be valuable aids in getting timely access to the right guideline. Posters for wards and stickers or markers in medical records can be simple methods of reminding staff; e.g. to prompt staff to check that all post-myocardial infarction patients are discharged on aspirin and beta blockers. Guideline mouse-mats, desktop calendars, and computer versions that can be accessed via local intranet are more sophisticated methods (Figure 7.3). Guidelines can be incorporated into relevant referral forms to encourage compliance with referral requests, e.g. with radiology requests. Recommendations can also be incorporated into reports (such as laboratory or investigations) or referral letters to reinforce desired practice. Computerized decision support will become

---

Box 7.6   Five key points to consider for practice education events

1. Be clear about the messages you want to get across.
2. Start the session by asking what issues the audience want addressed – write them down on a flip chart to try to cover the most important.
3. Try to make the session as interactive as possible. The audience will learn more if they have the opportunity to participate.
4. Encourage the audience to consider real examples from their own practice. There is good evidence that people tend to learn best if the topic is important to the learner and when learning combines reflection with concrete experience.
5. Try to see the topic from your audience's point of view. This may be a very different perspective from your practice.

an increasingly powerful method of reminder as it allows prompts to be made at the same time as clinical decision-making (see Chapter 8).

7. *Audit and feedback* allow individual wards and departments to see how their own clinical practice matches up with recommended standards and subsequently to monitor change. This information on performance can be important to demonstrate weaknesses in practice that justify the need for local guidelines. This can be used in the educational and training events to link key messages with evidence about current practice. It can also provide the basis for evaluation of the guideline uptake (an aspect which is important if you are to be objective about the effectiveness of your efforts) and the sustainability of changes in clinical practice.

8. *Patients* themselves can be influential in encouraging health professionals to make the right decisions. Well-informed patients will know what treatments they should be taking and what standards of care should be provided. This is particularly true of patients with chronic diseases and younger, more empowered patients. It is worth considering strategies that target patients themselves, such as posters in waiting areas, messages in the local press or discussions with local patient organizations.

Different mechanisms will work for different individuals, so try to tailor local approaches using the above menu of methods. Try to be systematic in the approach to implementation – adopting a stepwise approach may allow the best use of limited resources available (Box 7.7). For example, you can record attendance at educational and audit feedback events to monitor

---

Box 7.7   Example of a multifaceted implementation strategy: the Bradford and Airedale/Calderdale and Kirklees implementation of National Guidelines (BACKING)

A project manager was appointed to coordinate and support the implementation strategy across two health districts. Contextual analysis was undertaken at the start of the project to identify barriers to and incentives for local guidelines, and to inform the implementation strategy.

A) Developmental interventions
Local consensus groups of relevant stakeholders, including clinical governance leads, managers and influential professionals from primary and secondary care, were convened to:

- obtain commitment and ownership to improve quality of care using guidelines
- adapt nationally recommended evidence-based guidelines into a summarized local context
- agree appropriate implementation strategies based on the evidence and contextual analysis.

B) Dissemination interventions
A stepwise approach to disseminating the guidelines was taken in order to provide the greatest coverage of health professionals from the limited resources available.

Step 1: Education meetings
An interactive approach was taken with small group discussions, problem-based learning, case histories and worked examples. Local opinion leaders were identified by the steering groups and given specific training about leading the meetings. Additional primary care

Clinical guidelines and changing clinical practice

education meetings were held where gaps in existing district or Primary Care Trust (PCT) provision were identified.

The aims of the education strategy were to:

- use existing education systems and events to promote the guidelines
- run additional local education events where gaps in existing district or primary care group provision were identified
- establish local, smaller 'interactive' discussion groups adopting a variety of teaching methods, rather than larger didactic sessions
- share local information and the expertise of local speakers
- provide events that were accessible, accredited and met the needs of the target audience.

Education sessions for doctors and nurses working in secondary care and across the interface of primary and secondary care were also held.

Step 2: Educational outreach visits
Where no GPs from a practice attended these educational meetings, the practice was contacted and offered an outreach visit. Practices accepting the offer were visited by the project leader, asthma facilitator or cardiac rehabilitation nurse, who detailed the relevant guideline to practice GPs and nurses.

Step 3: Postal dissemination
Guidelines and accompanying information were posted to all the remaining GPs and practice nurses.

C) Reinforcing interventions
- The guidelines were designed, piloted and presented in a clear and concise format to improve readability.
- Guideline reminders were developed for clinicians. These included desktop calendars, laminated posters and mouse-mats. Patient-mediated interventions were also developed in order to target users (e.g. waiting-room posters) and disseminated in conjunction with the steps outlined above.

A marketing strategy was developed which included: a tailored communication strategy to target health professionals through a variety of channels including internet and local intranets; involvement of users and patient advocate groups in the development of the guidelines and patient information; local media campaigns with the involvement of local celebrities, e.g. local premier league football team.

coverage. Where possible health professionals who do not attend should be offered a group or individual outreach visit by the audit/guideline facilitator or other relevant staff (e.g. consultant or specialist nurse). When this is not possible, and as a last resort, guidelines should be sent by post to the remaining health professionals.

The final stage of implementation should be to evaluate the process of change and learn any lessons from it. Has there been the desired change? If so what worked? If not, what were the barriers and how can they be overcome? Changing practice is an ongoing process that must be reflective and adaptable if it is to succeed. Evaluation can be through audit of guideline standards or more qualitative techniques of interviews with guideline users and developers.

An example of a local guideline for best practice for patients with dyspepsia and *H. pylori* in primary care is shown in Box 7.8.

Box 7.8   Evidence into practice: management of patients with peptic ulcers and dyspepsia

Background: Eradication of *Helicobacter pylori* is effective in healing the majority of peptic ulcers and preventing relapses. In many patients with ulcer disease this eradication may eliminate the need for long-term maintenance with acid-suppressing therapy. These drugs comprise one of the most expensive cost categories in the NHS drug budget and therefore there is great potential to improve patients' health at a reduced cost to the health service. This topic was chosen to promote the implementation of effective management of patients with dyspepsia and peptic ulcer disease.

Implementation methods: A combined approach which included the development of evidence-based clinical guidelines, audit and feedback, outreach visits, educational workshops, patient reminders and the development of patient information linked to the guidelines.

Impact: 229 (86%) general practitioners attended group or personal education and feedback sessions. 44 (44%) practices took part in the audit. 1306 patients with a diagnosis of peptic ulcers were identified from audit of records. Follow-up after 9 months was completed for 66% patients. 10% of patients with ulcers had been prescribed eradication therapy for *H. pylori* at baseline compared with 50% at follow-up. Patients who had been prescribed eradication therapy were more likely to be off treatment with acid-suppressing drugs compared with those who had not (71% vs 19.1%). Costs of the project were £140 per patient known to have been treated with eradication therapy.

LIMITATIONS OF GUIDELINES

Although there has been a surge in popularity of guidelines, there are a number of drawbacks to remember. Guidelines tend to be based on a diagnosis – a starting point that is rare in the messy and uncertain world of real-life clinical practice. They can rarely be relevant to all patients, and will often focus on the more technical side of health care rather than reflect what the patients consider as important. From a professional perspective there is the threat that they will limit clinical freedom and promote a 'cookbook' approach to medicine, although in reality most professionals welcome guidelines for their decision-making and recognize that guidelines are what they describe – guidance rather than dogma. No one would describe the pre-flight checklist that airline pilots use as promoting 'cookbook' flying.

Some clinicians have concerns about the legal status of guidelines and fear being sued for non-compliance. However, the common legal measure of standards of medical care is that of customary practice that is accepted by a responsible body of doctors. This is called the Bolam test after a case of a man in the 1950s who fractured his pelvis during ECT and whose claim for medical negligence, on the basis of failure to use muscle relaxants during the procedure, was dismissed, because such practice was supported by a reputable body of medical opinion (see page 185). Adherence or non-adherence with guidelines is unlikely to prove decisive in cases of medical negligence unless the doctor's course of action strays from common professional standards.

One further potential weakness of guidelines is that they often concentrate on evidence of clinical effectiveness and rarely incorporate evidence of cost-effectiveness. This creates the potential for conflict between optimal and ideal health care. Cost implications of clinical recommendations must be considered if the guideline is to be successfully implemented and promote the greatest health benefit from limited resources.

CARE PATHWAYS

One way of encouraging adherence to guidelines or clinical standards is to build these recommendations and standards into the patient records. Typical medical records are unstructured and poorly completed. Different professionals tend to use different parts of the records and frequently ignore what their colleagues have written. This encourages haphazard documentation and much duplication.

Care pathways or integrated care pathways are health plans that describe the process of care from admission through to discharge for a particular condition, for example, myocardial infarction, stroke or particular surgical operations. They have a number of potential advantages:

- They can incorporate guidelines into records so that they act as prompts and reminders to health professionals.
- They highlight explicit standards to be met in the patient's pathway of care – standards that can be audited simply from the records to inform staff.
- They are multidisciplinary and so can improve communication between different professionals as well as cut down on unnecessary duplication of information recorded.
- They can reduce variation in clinical practice.
- They can improve documentation in health records.

The process of development of care pathways is just as important (and as time-consuming) as for guidelines. Spend some time identifying potential barriers to pathways adoption and avoid areas where there will be too much resistance. Choose a suitable clinical topic and convene a multidisciplinary team to develop the pathway. Standards and clinical prompts are then incorporated into a patient pathway and after piloting, reviewing and modifying the pathway, it can then be put into practice with an appropriate training programme for ward staff. Audit of records can then identify the degree of staff compliance and describe the common variations in care.

There is considerable experience in developing care pathways in different clinical areas in the NHS. Rather than start from scratch, try to identify suitable pathways that have been developed elsewhere. These can then be modified to fit the local context. An example of a care pathway is shown in Box 7.9.

Care pathways share some of the problems of guidelines. Like guideline development, the development of care pathways requires time, leadership and energy. They can become too inflexible and fail to take adequate account of the uncertainty of clinical practice. They may also stifle clinical decision-making by making it too automatic. Recording variations and deviations from the care pathway is important if these potential barriers are to be overcome and better pathways developed.

Box 7.9 Example of a care pathway for use in patients with a fractured neck of femur

FRACTURED NECK OF FEMUR PATHWAY

Patient Name: _____   A&E No. _____

Standards:	Init		Init
Patient to be fully assessed within 30 minutes of arrival at A&E	☐	Analgesic to be given within 30 minutes of arrival	☐
X-ray results within 60 minutes of arrival at A&E	☐	Arrival onto the ward within 2 hours of arrival at A&E	☐

	Day 1 A&E Date __/__/__ Arrival Time __:__	Init	Day 1 Ward Arrival Time __/__	Init
Clinical Assessment	Paramedic assessment Triage Nursing assessment Medical assessment Time pt fully assessed:__:__ Referral Ortho SHO Pain score Pressure area assessment		Hand-over – check A&E info Nursing assessment Medical assessment SHO – history and exam Consent Mark limb Request previous notes	
Clinical Management	IV opiate given Time given:__:__ Oral Diclofenac		TED stocking on both legs Fragmin (until mobile) unless contra-indicated Current medication prescribed Review pain management – pain score	
Radiology	X-ray results time:__:__ Pelvis X-ray Lateral of hip Chest X-ray		X-rays present on Ward	
Laboratory/ Investigations			Take bloods ECG in notes for theatre	
Hydration/ Nutrition	Peripheral venflon IV fluids if indicated		MQ assessment score Dietitian referral as necessary Oral care	
Communication/ Psychological Support	Assess and discuss with pt re: Diagnosis Plan of care Relatives present Relatives informed of above (if agreed by pt)		Assess and discuss with pt re: Introduction to ward/team Written patient information – Named Nurse – Visiting times – Diagnosis Relatives – discussion of above (if agreed by pt)	
Activity/Safety	Lifting and handling Observations T, P, R and BP Bed rest – assist with toileting		Pressure area risk assessment if water low 10 – core care plan Lifting and handling assessment Observations T, P, R & BP Hygiene Urinalysis Nurse-call system in operation Bed rest Assess sleep pattern	
Discharge Plan	Admitted from: Immediate home problems		Home circumstances assessment	

A DEVIATION FROM THE PATHWAY SHOULD BE DOCUMENTED IN THE PROGRESS NOTES

Signature of Named Nurse/Case Manager _____

Clinical guidelines and changing clinical practice

The development of electronic patient records will allow integrated care pathways to become electronic. This will ensure much greater flexibility and tailoring of prompts and standards to individual patients. It will also cut down on the excessive consumption of paper that generic care pathways tend to require. Electronic records are discussed in the next chapter.

FURTHER READING AND INFORMATION

Bero LA, Grilli R, Grimshaw JM, Harvey E, Oxman AD, Thomson MA. Closing the gap between research and practice: an overview of systematic reviews of interventions to promote the implementation of research findings. *BMJ* 1998; **317**: 465–468.

Cambell H, Hotchkiss R, Bradshaw N, Porteous M. Integrated care pathways. *BMJ* 1998; **316**: 133–137.

Dunning M, Abi-Aad G, Gilbert D, Gillam S, Livett H. *Turning Evidence into Everyday Practice*. London: Kings Fund, 1998.

Effective Health Care. Implementing Clinical Guidelines. University of Leeds, 1994.

Effective Health Care Bulletin. *Getting Evidence into Practice*. University of York, NHS Centre for Reviews and Dissemination, 1999.

Wensing M, Van der Weijden T, Grol R. Implementing guidelines and innovations in general practice: which interventions are effective? *Br J Gen Pract* 1998; **48**: 991–997.

Wright J, Bibby J, Hughes J. Evidence-based practice: Guiding Lights. *Health Service Journal* 1999; **109**: 30–31.

Communication, documentation and complaints

8

Good communication and recording of clinical information are the bedrock of good clinical care. Good communication is essential for patient understanding, consent and adherence to treatment. Good documentation is important for sharing information with colleagues and for defending actions when things go wrong.

This chapter deals with how we use and communicate clinical information in health care. This can vary from how well we talk to patients to the implementation of electronic patient records. The following topics are covered:

- Good communication
- Information provision: consent
- Good record-keeping
- Hospital coding
- Information for clinical decision-making: electronic records
- Accessing up-to-date clinical information.

GOOD COMMUNICATION

Good communication lies at the heart of all good clinical practice. This includes communication between health professional and patient, but also wider communication between health professionals in clinical teams and external communication, for example, with primary care, social services and other external agencies.

Poor communication is the cause of most complaints and litigation. Feedback from patients consistently highlights communication as a key priority in their perception of the quality of care they receive. Research studies have demonstrated that patients rarely feel that they have been given sufficient information by health professionals.

Good communication has been shown to:

- Improve patient adherence to treatment
- Increase effectiveness of treatment and outcomes
- Increase patient satisfaction
- Increase informed decision-making by patients
- Promote respect and empathy between health professional and patient.

With increasing consumerism and individual responsibility for health, demands for good, effective communication will continue to grow.

133

Good communication: 'You heard all wrong'

'If India's family planning policy has to succeed you all have a part to play.'

As final year medical students, all unmarried, from conservative backgrounds, even the most macho men in my class were beginning to wish that our project was something different, perhaps a nice nutrition study.

The teacher handed out oblong green coloured packets decorated with a red triangle, the family planning symbol. 'Go forth, convert the village, do your mite.'

We assiduously covered the 40 families we had been assigned, month after month, checking the empty containers and making sure that schedules were being followed.

In the fourth house, the woman hissed into my ear, 'I was due four days ago.'

I checked her packets and chart once more.

'Is the course completed?'

'Yes.' She nodded her head vigorously.

'Each time?'

'Yes. I am nauseated, and I want to eat only lime pickle.'

'Don't worry.' I patted her back reassuringly. Three months later there was a distinct bulge in the lower part of her abdomen. I escorted her back to the base hospital and consulted the professor.

'Sir, we were told that the pill was 99.9% effective. Her pregnancy test is positive.'

He pushed his spectacles up on to his bald pate and turned to the patient, 'Did you throw away the pills?'

'No, doctor.'

'Did you take them regularly?'

'No.'

I looked at her accusingly. 'You told me you had not missed a single dose.'

'No, doctor, you heard all wrong. I said that my husband did not miss a single dose.'

Gita Mathai *paediatrician, Vellore, Tamil Nadu, India*

(Reproduced with permission from: *BMJ* 2000; **320**: 1707.)

Good communication: 'Just my nerves'

Several years ago, before I permanently abandoned the clinic for the laboratory, I attended an elderly lady in the emergency department. She presented with 'chest pain', always a guarantee of early attention, but this chest pain was due to a band of haemorrhagic skin vesicles over the distribution of the fifth right intercostal nerve. They were exquisitely tender and there was adjacent hyperaesthesia. I examined her for evidence of lymphoma or other predisposing condition and found none. I told her that she had shingles, and explained that the chickenpox virus, often dormant from a childhood illness, spreads from the spinal cord out along the nerve, and that the nerve involvement was why the condition was so painful. I remember thinking that my explanation had been especially good. She nodded in understanding, and I explained that I would recommend some pain medicine, do some blood tests, and talk to her family doctor about her condition.

As I left the room, I told her husband, waiting outside, that he could go in. As he entered, I heard him ask, 'What did the doctor say?'

She replied, 'He said it was just my nerves.'

Jeffrey D Hubbard *pathologist, Albany, NY, USA*

(Reproduced with permission from: *BMJ* 2001; **322**: 278)

Barriers

Lack of time is a major barrier for all clinical staff. However, in view of the benefits of good communication this should not be an excuse. Opportunities should be made for alternative times or discussion with other team members.

Access can be a barrier. Clinicians should ensure that they are available to patients and their carers when necessary. Availability should be clearly stated. Language and disability can also act as barriers. Efforts to reduce these barriers, for example, through good access and use of interpreters, are vital.

Perhaps the commonest barrier is the belief that someone else will have told the patient or answered their questions.

Good practice

The following 11 points provide the foundation for good communication. Some may be obvious, but experience demonstrates that we often fail on the obvious.

1. *Introduce yourself by name and title*
2. *Assess what the patient understands and believes*
3. *Avoid jargon and technical words*
4. *Pitch at the appropriate level – use short words and sentences*
5. *Structure your conversation so that important information is given at the start and the end*
6. *Emphasize and repeat important information*
7. *Use a structure to communicate information (firstly, secondly…)*
8. *Give specific rather than general health advice*
9. *Maintain eye contact rather than looking at notes, and try active listening*
10. *Provide readable leaflets for written back-up*
11. *Document what you have told the patient.*

Two of the biggest omissions in communication are our failure to adequately *listen* and *understand*. Communication should be timely, accurate, sensitive and consistent. Privacy for the patient and relatives is crucial.

Standards

We are happy to define and apply standards for clinical practice but rarely consider doing so for such fundamental issues as communication. However, if we are to demonstrate improvements in quality of communication then it is essential to define standards. Examples of such standards are included below, along with audit criteria so that these standards can be measured and monitored over time. More sophisticated monitoring by using discharge questionnaires for patients at regular intervals should be considered.

Accessibility to medical staff

Standard: Medical staff are available to discuss diagnosis, treatment and prognosis with carers.

Satisfaction

| Satisfaction |

Satisfaction

Short waiting time
Be friendly rather than
business-like
Listen to patient
Find out what worries are
Find out what expectations are
– if not to be met say why

Content

| Selecting content |

Content

What does patient want to know
What are the patient's health
beliefs:
  Vulnerability
  Seriousness
  Effectiveness
  Costs and barriers

Understand /Memory

| Understanding and memory |

Understand /Memory

Avoid jargon
Use short words and short
sentences
  Simplification
Encourage feedback
Increase recall
  Primacy
  Stressed importance
  Explicit categorization
  Specific rather than general
  Repetition
Written back-up
  Readability

Fig. 8.1 Good practice in communicating with patients. (Adapted from: Ley P. *Communicating with Patients*. Croom Helm, 1988.)

Notes: All wards should have a policy to ensure that nursing staff can make arrangements for carers/relatives to speak with medical staff. This may occur on set days (e.g. following ward rounds) or at set times. However, flexibility will be required so that medical staff are available to discuss more urgent concerns with patients and carers.

Audit:

- Ask six sets of visitors on a given day
- Ask two members of staff on duty

Documenting communication of diagnosis, progress and treatment

Standard: Important information given to carers about diagnosis, prognosis and treatment is documented.

Notes: Communication with carers should be documented in the nursing kardex, whether by medical, nursing or therapy staff.

Audit: Check six case notes at random.

Private area for communication

Standard: All wards have a designated private area for counselling or discussion.

Notes: This may be a separate room, or office, where privacy can be guaranteed.

Audit: Ask staff on duty on the day of the audit.

Information on discharge

Standard: All patients are provided with information about their drugs and diagnosis on discharge.

Notes: Patients should be aware of the diagnosis and nature of medication at time of discharge. This may be via verbal communication, or preferably, simple written information.

Audit:

- Check the discharge of patients on that day.
- Check with ward pharmacist whether involved.
- Ask patients if anyone has been through the discharge letter with them.

Liaison workers and interpreters

Standard: Interpreters are readily available for non-English-speaking patients and patients with hearing impairment.

Notes: All wards should have a policy on communication with non-English-speaking patients; this may be via the hospital interpreter service or by ensuring that English-speaking family members are present (e.g. during ward rounds).

Audit: Check case notes of all appropriate patients.

Information leaflets

Standard: A range of written information is available to educate patients and carers.

Notes: All wards should either have, or know where to get, written information on common medical conditions (e.g. heart attack, stroke), social services provision and voluntary organizations; ward staff should be aware of which leaflets are available in the Trust.

Audit:

- Ask four members of staff what information is available (medical, social, relevant associations) on the ward.
- Review of notice boards.

CONSENT

Valid consent should be obtained from all patients as part of the routine process of good quality care. There is a legal and moral obligation for doctors to ensure that consent precedes any physical examination, surgical or medical treatment. Failing to obtain valid consent can result in litigation or complaints, as well as damage relationships with patients and undermine adherence to treatment. It is noteworthy that where issues of consent precipitate litigation it is often in cases of cosmetic surgery with no serious clinical outcome rather than life-threatening operations with serious clinical outcomes.

In the past consent has often been viewed as a signature on a form or a ticking of a box. However, consent is a process of discussion and information provision that results in the patient understanding the risks and benefits of examinations or treatments and giving their agreement. For consent to be valid, it must be provided voluntarily by an appropriately informed person (or parent of a child) who is competent to give consent.

For children, consent must be given by someone with parental responsibility; however, a competent child who consents to treatment cannot be overridden by a parent's refusal. Older children who fully understand what is involved in the examination or procedure can give consent themselves, although parents should be involved for under-16 year olds. When an adult is not competent to give consent, then treatment can still be given if it is in the best interest of the patient. These best interests should include the patient's needs and preferences, not just the medical interests, and carers may be able to provide valuable advice to inform this process.

There is no legal obligation to obtain written consent in the form of a signature, the traditional consent form merely reflects the prior discussion and information provision that has taken place over weeks and months. This process starts from the time the patient attends their general practitioner and subsequent outpatient appointment, to the time of the intervention. Patients should be able to change their mind at any stage before or during a procedure or treatment course.

Consent is essential for all of the 25 000 operations undertaken every day in the NHS, but is not something that is confined to surgical operations. Consent should be sought for all examinations and procedures. These include clinical examination, radiological investigations, blood tests and clinical photographs. Such consent may often be verbal rather than written.

When obtaining valid consent it is essential to determine what patients know, as well as their needs and wishes. As with all good communication, listening is the most important skill required before starting to provide patients with appropriate information. This information should include:

- The purpose of the investigation or treatment
- Explanations of the diagnosis
- Options for treatment, including the option not to treat
- The potential benefits and chances of success for different options
- The risks and side effects of different options
- A reminder that the patient can change their mind at any time
- Truthful answers to patients' questions.

The clinician providing treatment or investigation is responsible for ensuring that valid consent is obtained from the patient. Ultimate responsibility lies with the consultant, although the task of seeking consent can be delegated to

---

Consent: Always double check

The staff in the accident and emergency department had asked for a medical opinion on the first patient of the evening. Recently arrived from west Africa, the unfortunate young man was struggling to describe his numerous symptoms to his family in French, who were then translating his problems into English. I knew that this was not going to be straightforward.

Raised voices and increasingly frustrated gestures between the patient and his bewildered uncle and mother indicated that there were other issues at stake besides his fever, lethargy, and joint pains. After exhaustive questioning, I thought that a recent onset of dysuria was, perhaps, relevant in the aetiology of his problems. Although he emphatically denied any recent sexual contact, I wondered if this was more to do with the presence of his family members. Unfortunately, as it was late in the evening, there were no other translators available.

Sitting in front of the results computer later in the evening, I typed in my enigmatic patient's name and duly noted the normality of the tests that I had requested. As I pondered the differential diagnoses, I scrolled idly back through the results file, looking for any previous investigations. And there it was. Two days ago a urethral swab was sent from the genitourinary medicine department taken from my patient. I clicked on the relevant line to view the result – culture had grown *Neisseria gonorrhoeae*.

I returned to the cubicle and asked the patient's mother to wait outside. Through his uncle I asked the patient why he had been to the clinic two days before. He started to get angry, insisting that he had been nowhere near the clinic and that he could not have a sexually transmitted disease. He and his uncle exchanged words, and his uncle then asked if we could speak alone.

Out in the corridor the uncle explained that it was actually *he* who had attended the clinic earlier in the week and that he was currently taking antibiotics for gonorrhoea. He and the patient shared the same, albeit unusual, name and it was actually his result that I had seen and mistakenly ascribed to his nephew.

Having diagnostic information available without a patient's consent carries with it a degree of responsibility to check the accuracy and relevance of the information. Something I shall endeavour to do in future.

Lloyd Bradley *senior house officer in medicine, London*

(Reproduced with permission from: BMJ 2000; **321**: 1510.)

Communication, documentation and complaints

other health professionals who are suitably qualified and trained, with sufficient knowledge and familiarity of the procedure and the risks involved to inform the patient adequately.

In law the criterion used to judge the adequacy of information provided is the same as that used for assessing medical negligence (the 'Bolam test' – see Chapter 7), although the courts are the final arbiters of what constitutes responsible practice.

For the NHS, four model consent forms were introduced in 2002 to provide a consistent and recognizable form for patients and professionals (*www.doh.gov.uk/consent*). These cover consent for treatment for patients able to consent themselves; parents consenting for children and for adults unable to consent themselves. Accompanying these are information leaflets for patients about consent and also advice about the importance of backing up verbal information with written information about procedures. All doctors should read the patient information leaflets so that they are aware of what patients have been told and avoid the embarrassment of knowing less about patient rights than the patient.

GOOD RECORD-KEEPING

Good record-keeping is an essential part of maintaining quality of care. Health care records provide the reference point for different clinicians from different departments and disciplines. If information is incomplete or missing then the patient's life may be endangered. The records also provide the reference for medico-legal cases, and when, as so frequently occurs, there is no documentation describing the process and outcome of clinical care, there is no evidence that anything was done at all. If something goes wrong then there will no basis for defence in court.

Medical records also provide the basis for clinical coding so that diagnoses and treatments are coded and collated. This provides us with valuable information on clinical activity and outcomes. If the information in the medical records is not accurate then the coding and subsequent summaries of clinical work will be worthless.

The main point to remember is to keep medical records *accurate, legible and up to date.*

- Progress notes should be written every day or more frequently as events dictate.
- Each entry should be timed and dated and have the doctor's name and designation clearly printed after the signature.
- Abbreviations should be avoided.
- Abnormal results should be recorded.
- Details of information given to patients should be recorded.
- Diagnosis should be clearly recorded with the plan of management.
- Consent forms should be properly completed and signed.
- Discharge letters should be prompt and accurate.

Remember: *if it isn't documented, it didn't happen*

> **Box 8.1   Case example: arthroscopy**
>
> A man was admitted for arthroscopy of both knees. A nurse noted on the admission form that the patient had a previous history of thrombosis but this information was not entered on the operation form, which had a section for risk factors and known allergies.
>
> Before the operation the anaesthetist saw the patient and reviewed the operation form, but did not record whether the patient had told him about any previous episodes of thrombosis.
>
> The arthroscopies were carried out without incident and the patient was discharged from hospital later the same day. Two days later, he was admitted to the intensive care unit of another hospital with a pulmonary embolus arising from a deep vein thrombosis.
>
> A letter of claim from the patient's solicitors alleged that both the nursing and medical staff had been negligent in not initiating anticoagulant therapy postoperatively. The hospital agreed an out of court settlement for a clearly indefensible case with MPS contributing a small percentage on behalf of the anaesthetist.
>
> ---
>
> (Adapted from: *MPS Casebook*, Case Report, Issue 13, Summer 1999. Leeds: Medical Protection Society)

CODING

Hospital coders are a forgotten tribe. They trudge around the hospital wards unsupported and without acknowledgement. They live in basement cellars and broom cupboards and crave for the sunlight of recognition that rarely shines. Nobody believes their figures.

Yet it is their codes that form the basis for all hospital statistics. These hospital statistics are the foundation for all external assessment of quality and efficiency of health care within each hospital. In North American hospitals coders are well paid and have the best offices. They are the ones who are responsible for recording the activity and thereby the income of a hospital. Accuracy of coding is essential to obtain reimbursement and so the coders are valued and rewarded.

We are unlikely to see such a coding utopia in the NHS because the link between activity and funding is weaker. However, we need accurate and trustworthy information to review and audit our clinical activity such as frequency of diagnosis, case-mix, length of stay and outcomes.

Trying to improve coding can appear a Herculean task. While it may simply be a matter of junior medical staff documenting accurate diagnoses in the medical records, this is easier said than done. Encouraging consistency and accuracy of such documentation in a group of professionals who have a high turnover is an endless labour.

There are ways of improving coding, and it is worth pursuing the following ideas to achieve hospital information that is of use for monitoring quality and activity.

1. Discharge letters are often more accurate in diagnosis and procedures
   than the case notes. Copies of discharge letters should be considered as a

primary source of coding, although delays in their despatch often prevent this. They can also be used to validate what is coded from the case notes.

2. Improvements in the accuracy of discharge letters could be made if all patients received a copy of their own discharge letter. This would also improve patient access to medical record information and lead to more informed patients.

3. Greater awareness about the importance of coding should be promoted through providing educational slots during departmental clinical governance meetings. Staff from the coding department could then discuss problems with clinical staff.

4. Junior medical staff should be encouraged to peer review case notes from other departments. This raises awareness about weaknesses in documentation and acts as an incentive for better documentation in the department being reviewed.

5. Decentralization of coding staff to individual clinical departments could lead to better communication and closer involvement. Coders can then liaise with medical secretaries to ensure accuracy of coding.

6. Coders are often very skilled at gleaning information from poorly kept records, for example, by diagnosing hypertension from the patient's drug treatment. However, it is important to ensure that coders receive good support and training.

INFORMATION FOR CLINICAL DECISION-MAKING: ELECTRONIC RECORDS

As much as 25% of a doctor's time is currently spent chasing paper and results. It does not take too many sets of case notes to demonstrate that our traditional methods of record-keeping are inefficient, inaccurate and inaccessible. Over the next few years electronic patient records (EPRs) will be introduced in the NHS. These have the potential to revolutionize the quality of care we provide. Patient information will be accessible at any time and in any clinical location. Use of electronic records will improve legibility and completeness of medical records and potentially make them more secure. Results of laboratory and radiological investigations will be available at the clinicians' fingertips.

EPRs hold great potential to improve the quality of clinical decision-making and to monitor outcomes accurately and routinely. Clinical decision support can be integrated into electronic records, so that clinicians are provided with alerts and reminders. This can include:

- Prescribing support. When drugs are prescribed and recorded, decision support systems can prompt alerts to indicate drug interactions, allergies or wrong doses. These can help to reduce common prescribing errors.
- Clinical reminders. Electronic prompts can remind clinicians to document important information and to ensure that appropriate checks are performed. The record of a patient with diabetes in outpatients can remind the doctor or nurse to check the peripheral pulses and renal function.

- Referral guidelines. When a diagnosis is entered onto a record then this can prompt the integration of appropriate referral guidelines or treatment recommendations. This can form the first step of an electronic care pathway.
- Clinical requests and results. Electronic ordering of tests and services, including non-clinical services such as transport. Electronic access to lab tests and radiology results.

EPRs also hold great potential for monitoring the quality of care. With the routine recording of information about the process of a patient's care as well as health outcomes, collation of such information for audit and feedback of

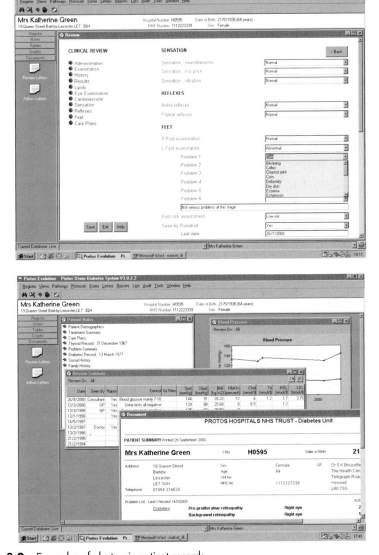

Fig. 8.2 Examples of electronic patient records.

Communication, documentation and complaints

clinical performance becomes a doddle. Gone are the tedious and time-consuming searching and trawling through patient case notes for frustrating audits.

The next stage after EPRs will be electronic health records (EHRs). Rather than having an EPR in place of hospital records, the EHR will provide a cradle to grave electronic record for patients wherever they are in the health and social care services.

This brave new world of paperless records is already in place in some settings in the NHS. The rest of us will follow with time. However, the solution is not just about information technology and clever software systems. The systems will only be as good as the people who use them, and to achieve appropriate use, recording and coding will require an ongoing programme of training and development.

ACCESSING UP-TO-DATE CLINICAL INFORMATION

The days of medical libraries, librarians and paper being our sources of information are coming to an end. These days we have knowledge centres and knowledge managers, worldwide webs and intranets. Rather than becoming an elephant's graveyard for research evidence, medical libraries are seizing the opportunities that electronic access provides for clinicians. Librarians themselves are developing their roles as knowledge managers rather than book filers. In these days of information overload their expertise in navigating the information highways and filtering out the rubbish is becoming increasingly important. Health professionals often do not have the skills or the time to access the appropriate information.

In the past, evidence about best clinical practice was scattered far and wide in a myriad of biomedical journals. Library databases such as Medline and Embase provide huge numbers of published papers (of variable quality), although finding the right papers is highly dependent on the quality and rigour of your searching skills. These databases are only able to provide summary information and abstracts rather than full text papers. However journal publishers are starting to provide greater access to on-line full text papers. The availability of these papers depends on whether or not your hospital or organization subscribes to the journal or portfolio of journals.

As the knowledge mountain has grown bigger and less accessible over time, clinicians have increasingly turned towards more user-friendly sources of knowledge and information. Although there is no single, comprehensive source of evidence, a number of summary resources are now available; for example, the Cochrane Library (Figure 8.3), Clinical Evidence (Box 8.2) and the Database of Reviews of Effectiveness. These are discussed elsewhere. The NHS also has its own on-line resource – the National Electronic Library for Health.

The National Electronic Library for Health (*www.nelh.nhs.uk*) is an on-line library for health professionals, patients and the public (Figure 8.4). It aims to provide a reliable source of accurate and up-to-date evidence about health

SELECTED: UNSELECT   SAVE   VIEW

- ▸ **The Cochrane Database of Systematic Reviews (2557)**
- ▸ **Database of Abstracts of Reviews of Effectiveness (3646)**
- ▸ **The Cochrane Controlled Trials Register (CENTRAL/CCTR) (348740)**
- ▸ **The Cochrane Database of Methodology Reviews (13)**
- ▸ **The Cochrane Methodology**

2002 Issue 3
ISSN 1464-780X

the cochrane library

the best single source of reliable
evidence about the effects of health care

The Cochrane Library presents the work of the Cochrane Collaboration and
others interested in assembling reliable information to guide health-care
decisions.

About the Cochrane Library

Using The Cochrane Library

Comments and feedback

Technical support

Fig. 8.3 The Cochrane Library.

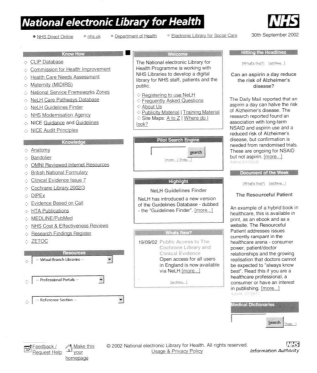

Fig. 8.4 The NeLH home page.

Box 8.2 Example of a summary from *Clinical Evidence*

Key Messages

Relapse rates and disability

- We found no evidence that any treatment alters long term outcome in multiple sclerosis (MS).
- Large RCTs in people with active relapsing and remitting MS have found that interferon beta-1a/b reduces relapse rates by a third and may delay development of neurological disability.
- One RCT in people with secondary progressive MS found that interferon beta-1b delayed development of disability by 9–12 months.
- One systematic review of RCTs has found that azathioprine has a modest effect on relapse rates.
- Evidence from single RCTs suggests modest benefit from glatiramer acetate, intravenous immunoglobulin (Ig), and methotrexate.
- Limited evidence from small RCTs suggests that pulsed intravenous mitoxantrone improves outcome in people with very active MS, in whom the risk of severe neurological disability may outweigh the risks of cytotoxic treatment.
- We found insufficient evidence about the effects of plasma exchange on neurological disability.
- We found no evidence about the effects of corticosteroids on long term outcome.

Fatigue

- One short term RCT found that amantadine modestly reduced MS related fatigue. It found no evidence of a benefit from pemoline.
- We found insufficient evidence on the effects of behavioural modification therapy or exercise in people with MS related fatigue.

Spasticity

- Two RCTs have found that tizanidine reduces spasticity in people with MS.
- We found insufficient evidence on the effects of other oral drug treatments or of physical therapy in people with MS related spasticity.
- One small RCT found benefit from intrathecal baclofen in non-ambulant patients with symptomatic spasticity resistant to oral drug treatment.

Multidisciplinary care

- Limited evidence from two RCTs suggests that 3–4 weeks of inpatient rehabilitation results in short term improvements in disability, despite no evidence of an effect on neurological impairment. The duration of this effect is uncertain.
- One small RCT found that prolonged outpatient rehabilitation reduced MS symptom frequency and fatigue.

(From: Ford H, Boggild M. Treament of multiple sclerosis. *Clinical Evidence* 2001; 5: 894–905.)

and health care. The NeLH is currently divided into 'floors', including a 'know-how' floor and a 'knowledge' floor, as well as Virtual Branch Libraries. The 'know-how' floor links to the National Institute for Clinical Excellence (NICE) guidance on systems of care, and National Service Frameworks. The 'knowledge' floor provides access to library sources such as the Cochrane Library, Clinical Evidence, Health Technology Assessment reports and national clinical guidelines. There is access to 'Virtual Branch Libraries' that specialize in topics such as cancer, mental health and diabetes. A search engine for locating relevant clinical information from across knowledge sources and databases is also included. Health information for patients is accessed through NHS Direct Online.

COMPLAINTS AND LITIGATION

Poor communication is the commonest cause of complaints, whereas poor documentation is the commonest problem in litigation cases. Tackling both of these areas will reduce complaints and unnecessary legal claims, but much still needs to be learnt from these surrogate markers of poor quality care. Rather than concealment and denial, we should treasure every complaint as an opportunity to find out how we can improve the quality of care that our patients receive, and to reduce the chance of future patients suffering.

Few doctors these days will escape from dealing with complaints and litigation, and the stress and anxiety they create for both patient and professional. The general public are increasingly demanding and vocal about the care they receive and it is hard to imagine patient expectations going anywhere other than upwards.

When patients complain they have three main reasons:

1. They want to make their view known and their voice heard.
2. They want an honest explanation and a heartfelt apology.
3. They want to ensure that it does not happen to others.

Some will have other reasons of revenge or financial gain, but these are the exceptions. By addressing these common reasons we can reduce the stress and anxiety for patient and professional and prevent the complaint from becoming a legal claim.

Dealing with patient complaints starts with the systems for making complaints in an organization. In the past these have often been labyrinthine and obstructive. There can be few greater incentives for patients to pursue complaints through alternative avenues such as legally or through the Ombudsman than the frustration generated by such obstruction. Complaints systems should be easily accessible, simple and speedy. Patients should have ready access to information, in appropriate languages, about how to complain. Their complaint should be dealt with seriously and impartially if it is to be resolved locally. Box 8.3 describes NHS complaints procedures.

The commonest causes of complaints are poor communication, staff attitudes and waiting times. The commonest themes that emerge from investigations are poor record-keeping, inadequate supervision and training, and weaknesses in handling complaints and dissatisfaction at an early stage.

From the doctor's point of view, there are two golden rules for dealing with complaints. The first is to give an honest explanation and an early apology. The majority of complaints will go no further if these simple steps are taken. The second goes back to the idea of every complaint being treasured, and that is to *listen* and *learn* from complaints in a department or a general practice. For this to happen effectively, organizations must have good systems to feedback complaints and their outcomes to individuals and teams.

Box 8.3   NHS complaints procedures

There is a two-stage complaints procedure in the NHS. The first stage is **local resolution**. This is the best opportunity for resolving complaints and will be successful in the majority of cases. Local resolution should be open and fair to both patient and professional.

If local resolution is not possible and the complainant remains dissatisfied they have the right to request an **independent review**. A local Convenor will assess the complaint and determine whether or not an independent review panel should be set up to try to resolve it. Many of the complaints that reach this second stage stem from dissatisfaction with the process of the first stage.

Complainants can at any stage refer their complaint to the Health Service Commissioner or Ombudsman. The Ombudsman will assess each case and undertake further inquiry and investigation into the complaint. Recommendations for change can be made to an organization in the light of an investigation. Only a small proportion of complaints end up with the Ombudsman, and the lessons and recommendations from investigations are often poorly disseminated to NHS staff.

FURTHER INFORMATION

Reference guide to consent for examination or treatment. London: Department of Health, 2001 (*www.doh.gov.uk/consent*).
Consent tool kit. London: British Medical Association.

Health outcomes and monitoring performance

'Measurement alone does not hold the key to improvement ... measuring could be an asset in improvement if and only if it were connected to curiosity – were part of a culture of learning and enquiry, not primarily of judgement.'

Donald Berwick

Quality improvement in the health service has traditionally relied on vague aspirations to do better next year. While the intentions have usually been good, the opportunities to demonstrate change and improvement have often been limited by the lack of goals and targets. These days governments are pre-occupied with targets and performance measures and the health service, as recipient of much taxpayers' money and political attention, has ended up with more than its fair share.

There is nothing new about measuring outcomes in health care. Florence Nightingale measured mortality in soldiers undergoing lower limb amputations and was able to demonstrate that death rates were higher in larger hospitals when compared with smaller hospitals. These days we can compare all the hospitals in the UK, and the amount of routine information available to us is huge.

This chapter describes how performance in the NHS is measured using national indicators, and then how individual hospitals are monitored through specific clinical indicators. The starting point for most of these indicators is usually what is currently being measured, rather than less tangible aspects of quality such as compassion and caring, so government health warnings are required.

PERFORMANCE INDICATORS

With the introduction of clinical governance has come the recognition that there is very little information available about the quality of care in the NHS. Finagle's Law describes the perverse situation whereby:

- The information you have is not what you want
- The information you want is not what you need and
- The information you need is not available.

This prompted the development of a national Performance Assessment Framework to help identify areas where the quality of care was poor and to allow the progress in improving quality to be monitored in the 280 hospitals and 100 health districts in the UK. This provides a form of 'benchmarking' to compare performance across the country.

The framework is a collation of statistics across a district or within a hospital, and may appear to be far removed from the practice of an individual clinician. However, they are important indicators of local health care and are being used increasingly by the media to judge hospitals and districts in league tables. Every clinician should understand what is being measured and what the implications are for local services.

Six key areas for monitoring have been included in the performance framework (Figure 9.1). Many of the indicators included in these six areas are repeated throughout. Their inclusion often relies more on the fact that they are routinely collected in the health service than because they are valid

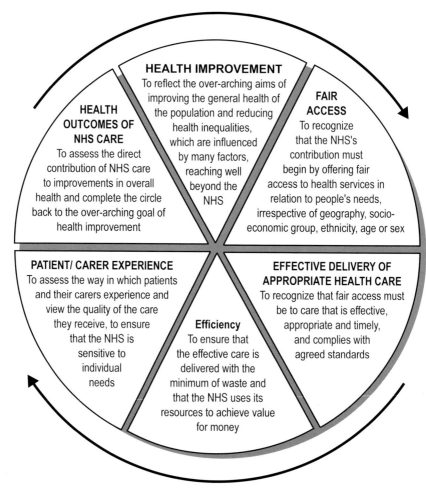

Fig. 9.1 The NHS Performance Assessment Framework.

markers of quality. The majority come from NHS datasets such as Hospital Episode Statistics (HES) or the Public Health Common Data Set.

1. *Health improvement.* This reflects the general aim of the health service to improve the health of the population. Many factors beyond the NHS influence the health of populations, particularly factors such as poverty and ethnicity. It is important to bear this in mind when making comparisons. Indicators include general death rates as well as specific priority areas such as cancer, heart disease and accidents that reflect the wider health status of the population:

   - Standardized all-cause mortality ratio (ages 15–64)
   - Standardized all-cause mortality ratio (ages 65–74)
   - Cancer registration rates – stomach, bowel, lung, melanoma, other skin, breast, cervix
   - Deaths from malignant neoplasms <75
   - Deaths from all circulatory diseases <75
   - Deaths from suicide
   - Standardized mortality rate from accidents.

2. *Fair access.* This measures the fairness of service provision in relation to need, geography, socio-economic status, age, sex and ethnicity. Indicators include:

   - Rates of surgery for operations considered to be very effective and where there may be a larger amount of unmet need, e.g. hip and knee replacement, cataract replacement, coronary artery bypass grafts.
   - Inpatient waiting lists to reflect variations in the supply and demand for services.
   - Registrations of adults and children with NHS dentists.
   - Early detection of cancer, e.g. percentage of women screened for breast and cervical cancer as a measure of access to screening tests.
   - Disease prevention – percentage of children immunized in a district.

3. *Effective delivery of appropriate care.* This is a measure of the extent to which local services are clinically effective, appropriate to local health needs, timely and in line with agreed evidence-based standards. Some are relevant to secondary care and include operations that are considered more effective (hip replacement) and those considered less effective (grommet insertion):

   - Discharge from hospital – within 65 days after emergency admission for stroke and 28 days after fractured neck of femur.
   - Inappropriately used surgery – age standardized D&C rates in women under 40 years, grommet insertion for glue ear.
   - Surgery rates – composite consisting of age standardized elective rates for coronary artery bypass grafts, total hip or knee replacement, cataract replacement.

   Some are markers of primary health care, such as hospital admissions of patients with acute and chronic diseases that should be avoidable, or poor prescribing:

- Acute care management – age standardized admission rates for – severe ENT infection, urinary tract infection, heart failure
- Chronic care management – age standardized admission rates for – asthma, diabetes, epilepsy
- Mental health in primary care – benzodiazepine prescribing
- Cost-effective prescribing composite – combination products, modified-release products, drugs with limited clinical value, inhaled corticosteroids
- Early detection of cancer – percentage of women screened for breast (50–64 years) and cervix (25–64 years)

4. *Efficiency.* This measures the extent to which the NHS provides efficient services, including cost per unit of care or outcome, productivity of capital estate and labour productivity. Indicators include:

- Day case rate as a marker of good resource use.
- Casemix-adjusted length of stay
- Unit cost of maternity services
- Unit cost of specialist mental health services
- Percentage of generic prescribing.

5. *Patient/carer experience.* This area covers the perceptions of responsiveness to individual needs and preferences; the care and continuity of service provision; patient involvement; good information and choice; waiting and accessibility. Indicators include:

- Waiting less than 2 hours for emergency admissions through A&E
- Operations cancelled for non-medical reasons on day of, or after, admission to hospital
- Delayed discharge for patients over 75 years old
- DNA rate for first outpatient attendance
- Percentage of patients seen within 13 weeks of GP referral
- Percentage of patients on waiting list for 12+ months.

6. *Health outcomes.* This measures the success of the NHS in using resources to reduce risk factors and levels of disease, impairment and premature death, and improvement in quality of life for patients. Indicators include:

- Emergency admissions in patients over 75 years old
- Emergency psychiatric readmission rates (a marker of community support)
- Infant mortality – stillbirths and infant deaths
- 5-year survival rates – breast and cervical cancer
- Avoidable mortality – e.g. from peptic ulcer, fractured skull, maternal mortality, TB, Hodgkin's disease, hypertension and stroke (in under-65s), asthma, appendicitis, cholelithiasis, cholecystitis, abdominal hernia, coronary heart disease in the under-65s
- Hospital deaths after surgery or heart attacks
- Dental decay in 5 year olds

Health outcomes and monitoring performance

- Conceptions in girls under 16 years
- Adverse events/complications of treatment – hernia recurrence rate, 28-day emergency readmission

CLINICAL INDICATORS

The performance framework includes indicators that will be influenced by many more factors than simply clinical care and, although it may be useful to gauge the quality of local health services, it may also appear to be rather irrelevant to most clinicians. However, a number of clinical indicators have been defined to try to draw attention to variations in outcomes across the country. These are a subset of the performance indicators listed previously, but can be considered separately for use by hospitals.

- Deaths in hospital within 30 days of surgery: emergency and non-emergency admission
- Deaths in hospital within 30 days of emergency admission with a hip fracture (neck of femur) for patients aged 65 and over
- Deaths in hospital within 30 days of emergency admission with a heart attack (myocardial infarction) for patients aged 50 years and over (Box 9.1, Figure 9.2)
- Emergency readmission to hospital within 28 days of discharge from hospital
- Discharge to usual place of residence within 56 days of emergency admission from there with a stroke for patients aged 50 and over (Figure 9.3)
- Discharge to usual place of residence within 28 days of emergency admission from there with a hip fracture (neck of femur) for patients aged 65 and over.

A number of other indicators were originally considered but not included in the final list. These include adverse drug reactions, wound infections, hernia recurrence and re-operation after prostate surgery. These were dropped because of difficulties in data collection, definition and clinical value.

Box 9.1   Clinical indicator example: deaths within 30 days of a heart attack

The rate in a local hospital was found to be higher than the national average (9.8%) at 11.9% (43 patient deaths from 359 admissions). After case note audit, 17 records were found to be wrongly coded with patients dying from other conditions. The recalculated rate was 7.6% (26/342), i.e. below the national average. Review of these patient deaths highlighted gaps in the quality of service including: delays in patients calling the ambulance, delays in thrombolysis after arrival at hospital, patients not being put on aspirin and beta-blockers where these were indicated. An action plan was developed to address these gaps. This included a community awareness campaign, the development of nurse-led thrombolysis teams and a monthly mortality and prescribing audit by the cardiology team.

Health outcomes and monitoring performance

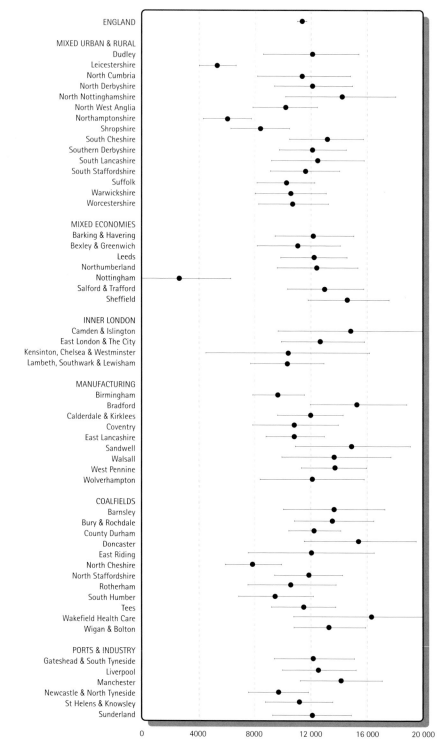

ENGLAND

MIXED URBAN & RURAL
Dudley
Leicestershire
North Cumbria
North Derbyshire
North Nottinghamshire
North West Anglia
Northamptonshire
Shropshire
South Cheshire
Southern Derbyshire
South Lancashire
South Staffordshire
Suffolk
Warwickshire
Worcestershire

MIXED ECONOMIES
Barking & Havering
Bexley & Greenwich
Leeds
Northumberland
Nottingham
Salford & Trafford
Sheffield

INNER LONDON
Camden & Islington
East London & The City
Kensinton, Chelsea & Westminster
Lambeth, Southwark & Lewisham

MANUFACTURING
Birmingham
Bradford
Calderdale & Kirklees
Coventry
East Lancashire
Sandwell
Walsall
West Pennine
Wolverhampton

COALFIELDS
Barnsley
Bury & Rochdale
County Durham
Doncaster
East Riding
North Cheshire
North Staffordshire
Rotherham
South Humber
Tees
Wakefield Health Care
Wigan & Bolton

PORTS & INDUSTRY
Gateshead & South Tyneside
Liverpool
Manchester
Newcastle & North Tyneside
St Helens & Knowsley
Sunderland

0   4000   8000   12 000   16 000   20 000

Age standardized rate per 100 00 and 95% confidence interval

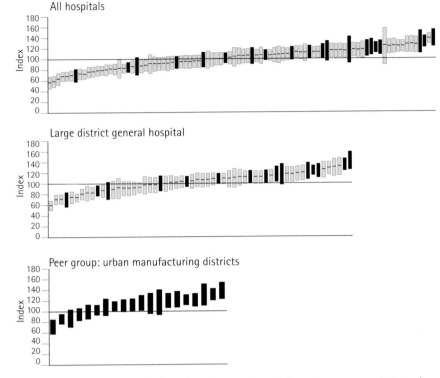

All hospitals

Large district general hospital

Peer group: urban manufacturing districts

Fig. 9.3 Discharge to usual place of residence within 56 days of emergency admission for patients aged 50 years and over with a stroke.

WHAT YOU NEED TO KNOW ABOUT CLINICAL INDICATORS

Clinical and performance indicators provide a starting point for open discussion about the quality of local services, but they must be interpreted cautiously and used not to cast judgements but rather to learn lessons. If they are seen as measures for allocating blame then they will quickly become discredited.

A number of issues need to be considered:

1. Do they improve care?
2. Data quality
3. Random variation
4. Casemix and comparisons
5. Sensitivity of indicators
6. Media reaction.

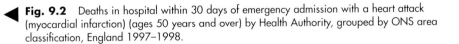

Fig. 9.2 Deaths in hospital within 30 days of emergency admission with a heart attack (myocardial infarction) (ages 50 years and over) by Health Authority, grouped by ONS area classification, England 1997–1998.

Improving care

The main reason behind publishing clinical indicators is to draw attention to poor performers so that they are prompted to examine the reasons why they come out worse than other hospitals and then do something about it. But do they really improve quality of care? The main experience of publishing this sort of information comes from North America. Although there were many concerns about data quality and casemix (see below), the publication of mortality data from certain operations did appear to reduce mortality over time, with clinicians learning from other hospitals about how health care could be improved. In addition, some surgeons who carried out few procedures with poorer outcomes stopped operating.

However, there are other outcomes that appear to happen with the release of this operative mortality data. Firstly, surgeons become more cautious about operating on high risk patients as they know that this may contribute to poor survival figures, even though it is often the case that the sicker patients have the most to gain. Secondly, there is more incentive to record co-morbidity to make the patients appear sicker and so justify higher mortality rates. This can lead to data manipulation and biased recording in attempts to improve league positions. Collecting information on patients who are operated on and those who are not would provide a fairer comparison of crude mortality data.

The clinical indicators for the NHS are broader than mortality rates for specific operations and less amenable to case selection and data manipulation. However, there will always be uncertainty over their role in improving care. While we are likely to see gradual improvements over time, this may be due more to improvements in data recording and case selection than quality of care.

Data quality

One of the first criticisms about the publication of clinical indicators was that the data they were based on were inaccurate. Few people would disagree with this and early experience confirmed that there was widespread inaccuracy in coding and classification of the hospital information that formed the basis for the indicators. For example, deaths following surgery were found to include 'surgical' procedures such as urinary catheterization and central line insertions. The first task that many poorly performing hospitals undertook was to review the quality of the information and ensure that in future years the information would be accurate. This is an important part of the process of improving care, as reliable and accurate information is an essential part of this type of benchmarking.

Random variation

Many of the outcomes recorded in the indicators are relatively rare events, e.g. deaths in patients with hip fractures. This means that a small number of deaths in a particular year can lead to large shifts in position in league table comparisons. This random variation will explain much of the variation between hospitals in any particular year and this should be borne in mind when examining the indicators. Confidence intervals can help to inform the significance of individual hospital results and it is important to consider trends over time rather than the results for one particular year.

Casemix

Comparisons between hospitals should be fair. For example, a hospital serving an older or poorer population could be expected to have higher mortality rates than one serving a younger more affluent population. Tertiary referral hospitals may be expected to have higher mortality rates as they take sicker patients from other referring hospitals. Some adjustment for differences in these patient groups (casemix) can be made by age and sex standardization of the clinical indicators. The other method that is used is to classify hospitals into comparable groups. The clinical indicators do this in terms of geographical and demographic variables such as urban, rural, coastal, manufacturing, coalfields and prosperous areas. In addition, hospitals are classified by type, e.g. small acute, large acute and acute teaching. This provides some equity in comparison, and not surprisingly, death and readmission rates tend to be higher in urban manufacturing areas than in rural prosperous areas.

A number of scoring systems have been developed to allow adjustment for casemix in surgical outcomes such as Acute Physiology and Chronic Health Evaluation (APACHE) and Physiological and Operative Severity Score for enUmeration of Mortality and morbidity (POSSUM) scoring system (Box 9.2).

Sensitivity of outcomes

The clinical indicators are meant to be measures of quality of care. However, they cover only a limited number of clinical areas, with a particular bias towards surgical specialties, and will be of no relevance to the majority of clinical specialties. In addition, they measure what is easily measurable – death, readmission and length of hospital stay. While these measures may represent a narrow and extreme marker of the quality of health care, they are far too crude to measure the many different components – from communication to environment – that define quality.

Each clinical specialty should consider developing outcome measures that they consider to be more accurate indicators of quality rather than relying

---

Box 9.2   POSSUM scoring system for surgical outcomes

POSSUM uses 12 physiological and six operative variables to provide a risk-adjusted assessment of morbidity and mortality. Observed to expected ratios (O/E) are calculated for individual surgeons or clinical teams and can identify where performance is below or above international standards for the operative procedure. Surgeons who operate on high risk patients thus have a valid assessment of their mortality rates that is adjusted for their casemix.

Health outcomes and monitoring performance

purely on what easily measurable outcomes are available. While this may be difficult (for example, how do you measure the amount of children's laughter that may reflect quality of care on a paediatric ward?) it provides a basis for understanding good patient care.

Examples of nationally developed outcome indicators for myocardial infarction and breast cancer are shown in Boxes 9.3 and 9.4.

Media reaction

The indicators are published for public consumption and there is inevitably a lot of interest in the press. The media have the difficult task of dealing with a large and detailed amount of information and turning it into easily digested newspaper articles. Their task is to sell papers and not to provide academic

---

Box 9.3   Outcome indicators for myocardial infarction

Indicators related to reduction of risk of a first myocardial infarction (MI)

1A*   Population-based heart attack rate for MI
1B*   Annual hospital admission rate for all MIs
1C   Annual hospital admission rate for first-ever MIs
2   Percentage of people who report having ceased smoking in the given year
3   Mean systolic blood pressure in persons aged 16 and over
4   Percentage of general practice patients, identified as hypertensive, whose most recent systolic blood pressure measurement is <160 mmHg
5A   Percentage of general practice patients identified as at high risk of coronary heart disease in the given year
5B   Summary of 12-month changes in the risk of coronary heart disease within a general practice population

Indicators related to reduction of risk of death from myocardial infarction

6   Population-based mortality rate from MI
7   Case-fatality rates for patients admitted to hospital alive with an MI
8   Proportion of patients attending hospital with MI who receive thrombolytic therapy
9A   Time from onset of symptoms to call for help
9B   Time from call for help to arrival at hospital
9C   Time from arrival at hospital to administration of thrombolytic therapy
10   Time from call for help to defibrillator availability

Indicators related to reduction of risk of subsequent myocardial infarction or other related cardiovascular events (*see below)

11A   Rate of inpatient admission for MI within 1 year of a previous hospitalized MI
11B   Rate of inpatient admission for selected cardiovascular conditions within 1 year of a previous hospitalized MI
12   Level of risk in respect of defined risk factors for CHD within a population of patients 6 months after first-ever MI

Indicators related to improvement of function and well-being after myocardial infarction

13   Impact of symptoms on function within a population of patients 6 months after first-ever MI
14   Assessment of health status/quality of life within a population of patients 6 months after first-ever MI

---

*1A and 1B are also related to the reduction of the risk of a subsequent myocardial infarction

---

Box 9.4   Outcome indicators for breast cancer

Indicators related to improvement of early detection and treatment of breast cancer
1A   Incidence of primary breast cancer by cancer stage at diagnosis
1B   Detection rate of small primary breast cancers
2   Incidence of interval breast cancers
3   Incidence of invasive breast cancer following treatment for ductal carcinoma in situ

Indicators related to reduction of death and complications from breast cancer and its treatment
4   Survival rates by cancer stage at diagnosis
5   Population-based mortality rates from breast cancer in women
6   Percentage of patients, diagnosed as having breast cancer, who had received a diagnostic triple assessment
7   Percentage of patients with breast cancer under the care of a breast care specialist
8   Percentage of patients receiving treatment for breast cancer whose care was planned jointly by a multidisciplinary group
9   Percentage of patients who, having undergone potentially curative surgery for breast cancer, were given chemotherapy as part of their primary treatment
10   Percentage of patients who, having undergone potentially curative surgery for breast cancer, were given radiotherapy as part of their primary treatment
11   Recurrence rates of breast cancer by site and type of primary surgery
12   Rates of specific complications detected, within 1 year of discharge from hospital, among patients having undergone inpatient treatment for breast cancer

Indicators related to maintenance of well-being during and following treatment for breast cancer
13   Delays from patient identification of symptoms to start of treatment for breast cancer
14   Patient satisfaction with specific areas of the management of their breast cancer care
15   Assessment of health-related quality of life within a population of patients 1 year after a diagnosis of breast cancer
16   Assessment of psychological distress in the patient following treatment for breast cancer
        A – measurement of psychological distress by use of an agreed instrument
        B – rate of referral to specialist psychological services

---

discussions on the information and so the headlines will always concentrate on the 'best' and the 'worst' and simplify into good and bad. So while Oxford may be described as the healthiest place to live and Manchester the sickest, there will be little explanation into the socio-economic differences that underlie this variation.

The attention of the national media will always be a major incentive for hospitals to ensure that they remain anonymously average rather than risk being picked on as a poorly performing outlier, and this highlights the problem of these indicators focusing on outliers and ignoring all the good work that may be going on in the majority of hospitals.

A more important consideration should be the reaction of the local press; they will have a genuine interest in the performance of local health services. Relationships between hospitals and local health reporters are usually good and this co-operation should provide the basis for responsible and informed reporting about local results.

HOW TO DEAL WITH CLINICAL INDICATORS

Clinical indicators should not become the focus of attention for monitoring performance. However, they are the main measure of hospital quality that the general public will read about and can highlight potential problems. A number of steps should be taken to ensure that the information is used constructively.

1. Each department for which there are relevant indicators (e.g. cardiology, surgery, orthopaedics, care of the elderly) should have a nominated individual responsible for clinical indicators.
2. The medical director (or other senior clinician) and director of information services should work closely with these individuals to review the clinical indicators for the hospital.
3. An audit of the quality of data should be undertaken to examine the number of cases that make up each of the rates used in the indicators and to check on whether there are any obvious coding errors or anomalies. The denominator used in the rate should also be checked for accuracy.
4. Each relevant department should review their rate a) for each individual consultant, b) over time and c) relative to other comparable hospitals and discuss reasons for variation in an open forum.
5. Where indicators suggest below-average performance, a full medical record audit should be undertaken for all the cases that make up the indicator. This should determine the accuracy of the coding information and the details of patient care for each case.
6. The relevant department should review the results of this audit in their clinical governance meeting, discuss reasons for gaps in quality of care and set up changes in systems to ensure that these gaps are closed. Prospective audit of relevant cases and development and implementation of clinical guidelines may support such changes.
7. Consider joining with other hospitals to compare performance in a benchmarking club. Some commercial organizations, such as CHKS, provide this benchmarking service for NHS hospitals.
8. It is worthwhile spending time with the local health reporters and ensuring that they are aware of the limitations of the indicators and how the hospital is dealing with them.

Although these performance indicators have been chosen nationally, and will receive more than their fair share of attention and enquiry, it is important that clinical staff choose performance indicators that the department will find useful. The rationale for performance measures should be learning rather than judgement, and local measures can help determine what changes are required and what changes work in improving care (see PDSA cycles in Chapter 2). These home-made indicators can be just as useful as those chosen nationally if staff in the department value them and they can be used to measure quality of care. They do not have to be constrained by cold science and statistics. The number of patients smiling during a ward round may be more of an accurate reflection of quality of care than length of stay, it is just harder to measure.

Teamwork

'We need to honour our teams more, our aggressive leaders and maverick geniuses less.'

R.B. Reich: Harvard Business Review, *1987*

This chapter looks at:

- Working in teams in a modern NHS
- Models of teamwork
- Characteristics of effective teams
- The quality aspect
- Communicating with colleagues
- Learning in teams
- The patient and the team
- Sharing decision-making
- Towards partnership
- Listening to what patients want
- When things go wrong.

WORKING IN TEAMS IN A MODERN NHS

Almost everyone who seeks medical care interacts with more than one health professional. In teams, performance depends both on individual excellence and how well people in the team work together. In a modern NHS, with medicine and health care increasing in complexity, high quality care for patients will increasingly depend on high quality teamwork, so the quality of clinical teams will be an important clinical governance issue. It becomes increasingly necessary to be sure that the skills of all health professionals are used to the full. Good care depends on effective collaboration between many people. This means working and learning in teams, but it does not mean relinquishing the key doctor–patient relationship, which is so central to the therapeutic process.

A great deal of health care is already delivered by multidisciplinary teams. It has been clearly shown for aviation that formal training in team management and communication skills can produce substantial improvements in human performance as well as reducing safety-critical errors.[1] Nowadays it is probably not possible to deliver all the responsibilities of modern clinical practice, including clinical governance, on one's own as an independent practitioner. However, in some medical teams such as those in operating theatres, interpersonal and communications issues have been shown to be responsible for many inefficiencies, errors and problems in what is a psychologically and organizationally complex environment.[2]

MODELS OF TEAMWORK

The concept of the team based on the traditional model of a hospital consultant with a pyramid of juniors[3] is changing to that of a modern clinical team or directorate. In the past the clinical team was often thought of as consisting of a consultant with a retinue of junior doctors of various grades, and nurses and others at their beck and call. Given the range of responsibilities and multiplicity of expectations now encountered, this is no longer sustain-

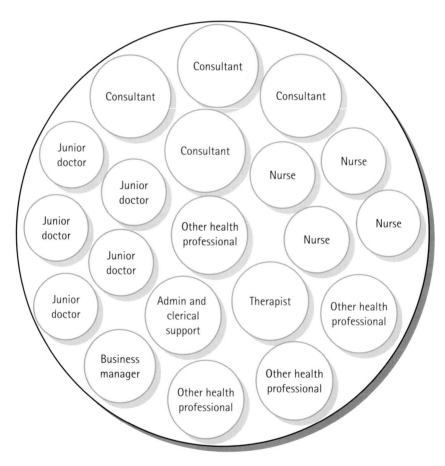

Fig. 10.1 The clinical team staffing resource.

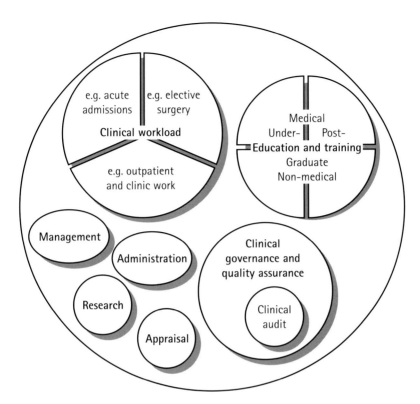

Fig. 10.2 The responsibilities of a clinical team.

able. Rather a clinical (or for that matter a general practice) team can be looked at in terms of its total human resource (Figure 10.1). This team then has to meet a whole range of responsibilities (Figure 10.2). A major part of these responsibilities is, of course, the clinical workload, with the nature and balance of clinical activity varying from team to team and specialty to specialty. But clinicians have other responsibilities too. The recent new responsibility for clinical governance is a corporate one. It is also one which overlaps with other responsibilities such as clinical audit.

CHARACTERISTICS OF EFFECTIVE TEAMS

There is a vast management literature on teams and team functions, group dynamics, team building and team management. In the NHS such groupings may exist within individual departments, within an organization as a whole, and now increasingly between organizations.

The most quoted study on roles argues that the most effective teams are not those containing the 'brightest and the best', but rather those which have a good balance between eight main roles.[4]

Teamwork involves different functions working together, and different people working together, so that each enhances the performance of the rest. The

a)

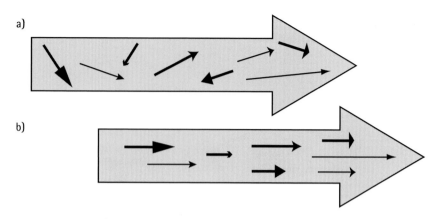

b)

Fig. 10.3 (a) Unaligned individuals in a team; (b) team members aligned in purpose and direction. (After: Senge PM. *The Fifth Discipline: The Art and Practice of the Learning Organization*. London: Random House, 1999.)

team can be a powerful influence in terms of changing its members' behaviour. Each function or specialization should seek opportunities to enable other functions or specializations to be more effective in the delivery of high quality patient care. Each person should seek to enable other team members to work out their individual strengths, especially when those strengths may be different. Alliances need to replace antagonism, with people making constructive use of differences. The whole can then be greater than the sum of the parts.

Team members need to be aligned in their purpose and direction (Figure 10.3). The fundamental characteristic of the relatively unaligned team is wasted energy. Individuals may work extraordinarily hard, but their efforts do not translate efficiently into team effort. By contrast, when team members become more aligned, they all pull in the same direction, and the energy of individuals harmonizes. There is less wasted energy, and indeed synergy may develop. There will be commonality of purpose, a shared vision, and an understanding of how to complement one another's efforts. Individuals do not sacrifice their personal interests to the larger team vision; rather, the shared vision becomes an extension or part of their personal visions.

Key features of teamwork include making the care of the patient the highest priority, and having respect for other people's knowledge and skills. In the past it has often been difficult for a doctor to accept that they may not necessarily automatically be the right person to lead a particular team. There has to be an acknowledgement of the legitimacy of other team members.

The characteristics of effective clinical teams have been well described (see Box 10.1).[5]

THE QUALITY ASPECT

Hand-over rounds between junior medical staff and all other groups of staff are a crucial component of care and risks reduction. Traditionally such hand-

---

Box 10.1   Characteristics of effective teams

Effective teams are teams which:

- show leadership
- have clear values and standards
- are collectively committed to sustaining and improving quality
- foster learning through personal and team professional development
- care for each member
- have a 'no blame' culture
- are committed to the principle of external review
- are open about their professionalism

Effective teams use:

- clinical guidelines and operational protocols
- good systems
- good data
- good records
- focused education and skills training
- systematic audit of performance with feedback
- regular, formative peer appraisal
- critical incident review
- risk management methods

(Adapted from: Irvine D. The performance of doctors. II: Maintaining good practice, protecting patients from poor performance. *BMJ* 1997; **314**: 1613–1615.)

---

overs have been part of nursing and midwifery practice, but not routinely part of medical practice. The pressures on and reductions in hours of work, and the introduction of various models of shift and other new patterns of working mean that it is incumbent on senior staff to insist and ensure that hand-overs are done effectively, seeking the resources (particularly time) that are required. Records, including clinical management plans, therefore need to be legible. There are also risks in this process. The clinician may fail to reassess a patient handed on by a colleague. There is also a danger of the perpetuation of an error made by the departing doctor or other health professional.

There is continuing tension between needing a minimum number of patients with particular clinical features or conditions, or undertaking a minimum number of a certain operation in order to maintain quality, and the desire of patients and communities to have easy access to every service. This means that clinicians have to link together to share experience and expertise, as well as expensive resources or facilities, e.g. magnetic resonance imaging. This is the thinking behind the concept of managed clinical networks.

The complexity of modern care means that not all units or teams can provide all services. The emergence of evidence that, for example, for many operations, minimum throughput numbers are required means that clinical networks are developing – teams of teams. Hub and spoke models of care, for example in the provision of cancer care, have been created (Figure 10.4). In such models, high level expertise, such as that available in tertiary centres, is linked functionally with a number of more locally based peripheral units.

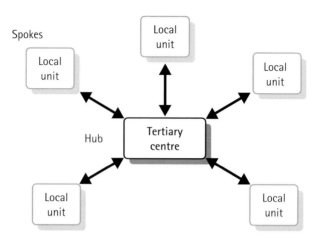

Fig. 10.4 Hub and spoke model of care.

Colleagues in these peripheral units can not only draw on the expertise available to them from a centre, but may themselves contribute to care at the centre. Therefore patients may get more coherent care, especially when complicated elements of care are needed, as in the diagnosis and treatment of cancers, which are only found in different locations. Professionals get a greater variety and number of clinical cases or experience, enabling them to maintain or enhance skills.

COMMUNICATING WITH COLLEAGUES

Medicine promotes sub-specialization to deal with the increasing intricacy of clinical care. Doctors end up retreating into their chosen field and links with other specialities can be weak. Clinicians working in a hospital will often know their speciality colleagues based hundreds of miles away better than they do their own hospital colleagues working down the corridor. One consequence of this dispersal of knowledge and skills is that clinicians lose touch with each other and end up bemoaning the lack of knowledge of their colleagues in other specialities or health sectors ('… if only they knew a bit more about my clinical field, then I would get fewer inappropriate referrals and unnecessary workload').

Effective communication is the key to overcoming such speciality isolation and siege mentality. A number of approaches to *outward* communication should be considered:

- *Clinical meetings*. These are the traditional forum for communication within clinical departments, but are underused for disseminating information between departments. In some areas, such as cancer care, multi-professional meetings are the norm, but the opportunity for such cross-speciality collaboration is often limited in other fields.

Box 10.2   Skills of a chairperson in meetings

- Focus on the agenda and meeting objectives
- Introduce new information appropriately
- Recognize when more information is needed to make a decision
- Clarify points of confusion
- Summarize the position reached
- Encourage all members to contribute
- Deal with difficult members and conflict
- Seek consensus
- Push the group to make decisions
- Find new ways round a problem

- *Divisional meetings.* These cover a wider number of related specialities with a greater business focus. Mutual trust, agreed objectives and shared expectations are all important components of effective meetings and should be established from the start. The right chairperson with the right skills is a prerequisite (Box 10.2).
- *Hospital meetings.* These may be clinical governance meetings or business meetings, but can provide a good forum for dissemination to a wider, if sometimes selective, audience. The potential barrier here depends on how well information is fed back to different departments.
- *Primary care trust meetings.* Most primary care trusts now have protected learning time or educational events for all practices or quality teams from different practices. Again the potential barrier to wider dissemination depends on how well the individuals attending communicate with their partners.
- *Workshops.* These can be great events for sharing good practice on a specific topic, as long as they are interactive and participatory. If the topic is important then it is easy to generate interest and attendance, although this may be rather selective from those already converted. The downside is the organization and administration necessary to run them, but the reward can be worth it.
- *Outreach visits.* Taking the message out to clinicians may be the only way to get to the hard-to-reach groups. The message can be tailored to the individual, and this form of communication can be very effective (which is why the pharmaceutical industry invests so heavily in it). However, it is time-consuming and expensive in terms of staff time.
- *Newsletters.* These can be an excellent method of spreading the word across a hospital or a district. Each department may develop their own, although this leads to an overload in mailings and a lot of work. Alternatively a hospital-wide newsletter can include sections from each department to spread good practice and disseminate information (Figure 10.5).

Communicating outwards is important to change others; however, communicating inwards is essential to understand what colleagues and patients want. Communicating inwards with colleagues can be as simple as using the frequently atrophied skill of listening. It can also take place through observing how care is delivered and how people work to identify gaps in care, or

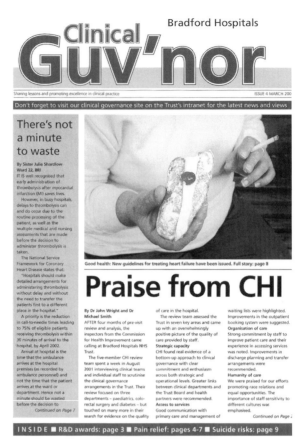

Bradford Hospitals

Clinical Guv'nor

Sharing lessons and promoting excellence in clinical practice   ISSUE 4 MARCH 200

Don't forget to visit our clinical governance site on the Trust's intranet for the latest news and views

There's not a minute to waste

By Sister Julie Shardlow
Ward 22, BRI

IT IS well recognised that early administration of thrombolysis after myocardial infarction (MI) saves lives.

However, in busy hospitals, delays to thrombolysis can and do occur due to the routine processing of the patient, as well as the multiple medical and nursing assessments that are made before the decision to administer thrombolysis is taken.

The National Service Framework for Coronary Heart Disease states that: "Hospitals should make detailed arrangements for administering thrombolysis without delay and without the need to transfer the patients first to a different place in the hospital."

A priority is the reduction in call-to-needle times leading to 75% of eligible patients receiving thrombolysis within 30 minutes of arrival at the hospital, by April 2002.

Arrival at hospital is the time that the ambulance arrives at the hospital premises (as recorded by ambulance personnel) and not the time that the patient arrives at the ward or department. Hence not a minute should be wasted before the decision to
Continued on Page 7

Good health: New guidelines for treating heart failure have been issued. Full story: page 8

Praise from CHI

By Dr John Wright and Dr Michael Smith

AFTER four months of pre-visit review and analysis, the inspectors from the Commission for Health Improvement came calling at Bradford Hospitals NHS Trust.

The five-member CHI review team spent a week in August 2001 interviewing clinical teams and individual staff to scrutinise the clinical governance arrangements in the Trust. Their review focused on three departments – paediatrics, colo-rectal surgery and diabetes – but touched on many more in their search for evidence on the quality

of care in the hospital.

The review team assessed the Trust in seven key areas and came up with an overwhelmingly positive picture of the quality of care provided by staff.

Strategic capacity
CHI found real evidence of a bottom-up approach to clinical governance with clear commitment and enthusiasm across both strategic and operational levels. Greater links between clinical departments and the Trust Board and health partners were recommended.

Access to services
Good communication with primary care and management of

waiting lists were highlighted. Improvements in the outpatient booking system were suggested.

Organisation of care
Strong commitment by staff to improve patient care and their experience in accessing services was noted. Improvements in discharge planning and transfer arrangements were recommended.

Humanity of care
We were praised for our efforts promoting race relations and equal opportunities. The importance of staff sensitivity to different cultures was emphasised.
Continued on Page 2

INSIDE ■ R&D awards: page 3 ■ Pain relief: pages 4-7 ■ Suicide risks: page 9

Fig. 10.5 An example of a hospital-wide newsletter: Bradford's *Clinical Guv'nor*.

through staff surveys to obtain feedback and views. Obtaining patient feed-back can be more complicated (see page 176).

LEARNING IN TEAMS

Most clinical teams are involved in one way or another with education and training. Most health professionals have at least one characteristic in common (a personal desire to learn), and they usually have at least one shared value (to meet the needs of their patients). The team must not only meet its own learning needs, but must meet the responsibility for educating and training the next generation of health professionals. Many teams now will be involved with undergraduate and postgraduate students, both medical and non-medical. For example, trainees need not only to learn the theory and principles of clinical audit, but also to see it done and used routinely in the everyday working of the team, and not as an add-on extra.

In meeting their own needs, teams will have to learn how to work with each other within the team, and with others outside. They will need to learn how to deal with conflict, and handle sensitive issues. They need clear goals, with built in feedback on performance.

It is logical that if doctors and other health professionals are to work together effectively in teams, then they must learn together in teams. This also requires practice. It would be inconceivable to expect an orchestra to play music well without rehearsals. Learning in teams is itself a skill.

The discipline of team learning involves mastering the practice of dialogue and discussion, the two distinct ways that teams converse. In dialogue, there should be the free and creative exploration of complex and subtle issues. This means listening to each other, and suspending one's own views. In discussion, by contrast, different views are presented and defended. There is a search for the best views to support clinical or management decisions that must be made. Dialogue and discussion should be complementary, but many teams lack the ability to distinguish between the two or to move freely between them.

Team learning must therefore involve finding ways to deal creatively with the powerful forces that prevent productive dialogue and discussion. This may mean avoiding attempts to smooth over differences, or perhaps a free-for-all where nothing is held back; both are defensive mechanisms that inhibit learning and effective teamworking.

Significant event analysis has enormous educational potential for developing professional practice. Significant events are those which occur, usually unpredictably, and lead to, or may lead to, adverse outcomes. The analysis is

Teamwork

Box 10.3   Guidelines for significant event audit meetings

- In general, cases chosen will have had a poor outcome or a 'near miss'
- It is not an appropriate technique where legal action is anticipated or where individual incompetence is suspected
- All the members of the relevant multidisciplinary group involved in the care should participate
- The aim is to be supportive to team members – all feedback should be constructive and not negative
- It is not an attempt to search for the 'right way', but a means of exploring possible alternatives for the future
- The chair (or external facilitator, if used) should not have been actively involved in the case under discussion
- A brief anonymized written summary of the case can be made available at the meeting, providing key dates and relevant factual information
- The case should be introduced by a brief presentation from the involved team member(s)
- The chair should compile a written summary of the general conclusions with any actions to be taken, for review at a future specified date
- The chair's summary should be the only record of the meeting
- Individual team members' actions in the care of the case and their contributions to its discussion at the meeting should not be discussed outside the meeting

---

(Adapted from: Clinical Governance in Primary Care. Adapted from: Robinson LA, Stacy R, Spencer JA, Bhopal RS. How to do it: use facilitated case discussions for significant event auditing. *BMJ* 1995; **311**: 315–318.)

Box 10.4   Role of the chair (or external facilitator if used) in significant event audit meetings

- To explain the aims and process of the discussion
- To structure the discussion – i.e. to keep to time, to encourage contributions from all participants, and to clarify and summarize frequently
- To maintain the basic ground rules of group discussion, for example, to allow uninterrupted discourse, to encourage participants to speak for themselves (using 'I' not 'we'), and to maintain confidentiality
- To clarify suggestions for improvement and identify who will be responsible for initiating change
- To recognize, acknowledge and enable appropriate expression of emotion within the group
- To remain 'external' to the group and to avoid giving unwarranted opinions or colluding with the group during discussions
- To compile a written summary of general conclusions with any actions to be taken, for review at a later date

(Adapted from: Clinical Governance in Primary Care. Adapted from: Robinson LA, Stacy R, Spencer JA, Bhopal RS. How to do it: use facilitated case discussions for significant event auditing. *BMJ* 1995; **311**: 315–318.)

designed to achieve learning about how things could be done better in future, and not to apportion blame. There are therefore strict rules for conducting such analyses, based on assessing the facts (see Boxes 10.3 and 10.4).

THE PATIENT AND THE TEAM

It can be argued that the patient should be at the centre of the team, and indeed any health care process. Indeed, the patient's need should drive the system. The future of medicine is not about robot lasers, gene therapy, miracle cures or tumour-seeking micro-computers. The future of medicine is far more mundane and fundamental. It is about promoting partnership with patients.

In recent years there have been trends in quality improvement in the health service, for example, teamworking, audit, evidence-based practice, risk management, clinical guidelines, R&D, health technology assessment. All are methods of improving standards and all have made their impact on clinical practice. All are important pieces of the clinical governance jigsaw.

Just as the old pyramidal hierarchical model of a consultant and his team providing care to patients can no longer be sustained, the modern clinical team cannot operate in isolation. In many cases the patient journey crosses a variety of thresholds and boundaries. Teams therefore need to communicate effectively with each other not only within hospitals and practices, but also between them. Examples of services and teams reorganized around the patient pathway through care and services are shown in Figures 10.6, 10.7 and 10.8. However, the next challenge is clear and over-riding, and that is ensuring the real involvement of health service users.

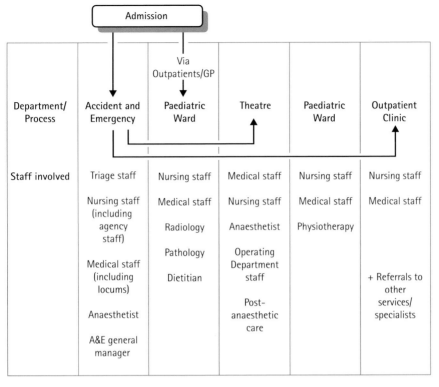

Fig. 10.6 A patient pathway in paediatrics.

PATIENT PARTNERSHIP

Involvement of users of health services has long been a neglected area. In the past it has often been considered unnecessary or irrelevant. More recently many health organizations have started to enhance their accountability through increasing user involvement, although this has frequently been cosmetic rather than any real attempt to ensure increased user influence.

Patient partnership: Patient empowerment

He was 62 years old, a teacher by profession, and had recently had hypertension diagnosed. Metroprolol had been started two weeks ago and his next appointment was not for another two months, but this morning he had insisted on being seen.

He sat demurely opposite me and, just as I finished reviewing his case history, looked straight at me and said, 'Doctor, I would like to have you know that for the past two weeks my corpus spongiosum has not been filling up adequately.'

I was stumped. For about 20 seconds, which seemed like an eternity, my mind was a complete blank. I have forgotten much of my medical school anatomy. And then, by a miracle, I remembered. 'Why don't you tell me you are not able to have an erection?' I asked defensively.

'I thought you doctors like to be technical,' he retorted without meaning to be impolite. 'Anyway, I read from the internet that metoprolol can cause impotence.'

Knowledge is power. The internet, that maze of information, is becoming available to increasing numbers of Malaysians. Many of my patients are getting a profusion of medical information from the internet, some of it accurate and some totally unreliable.

I am a firm and passionate believer in patient empowerment, but that particular morning the impact of knowledge and patient empowerment hit me like a ton of bricks. With that little discourse I realised that the internet has provided this patient with the knowledge that his recently acquired impotence was drug induced. Without this information, he would probably have considered his erectile dysfunction as a normal part of ageing and never mentioned it to his doctor. Instead, patient empowerment made him feel comfortable about 'confronting' his doctor with his suspicion, a behaviour that is not usual in Malaysian society, especially when the issue is sexual and so very personal.

I changed his antihypertensive medication. Two weeks later, he called to tell me that he had regained his sexual prowess. Had it not been for the internet and patient empowerment, an important aspect of his life would have vanished.

Today, when I run my clinic my computer is always on line in case a patient raises any query as a result of surfing the net, and when I explain anything to a patient I consciously use simple term so as not to be 'technical,' and sitting on my table is a message to my patients: 'Your health is as much your responsibility. Take charge.'

P H Chew *head of department of medicine, Sarawak General Hospital, Malaysia*

(Reproduced with permission from: *BMJ* 2001; **322**: 1472.)

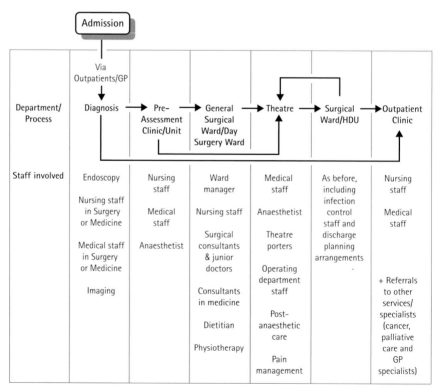

Fig. 10.7 A patient pathway in general surgery (focusing on colorectal surgery).

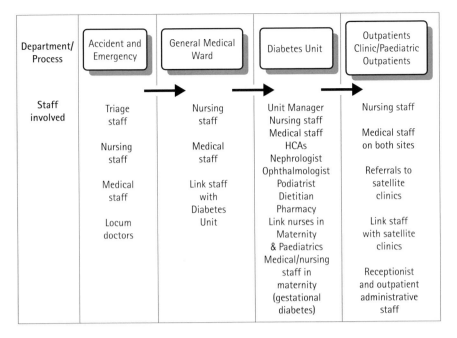

Fig. 10.8 A patient pathway for diabetes.

Any discussion about quality of care is meaningless unless it includes the perspective of the user. Doctors will often concentrate on the technical aspects of quality, such as surgical skill or complications. However, patients usually take these aspects for granted and are more concerned with quality issues such as communication, waiting times and the environment. The adage that the operation was a great success but the patient died reflects these different priorities.

If we are to take quality seriously then we need to begin and end with the user's perspective. This acknowledges the two key reasons for user involvement. Firstly as a **consumerist** approach to ensure that the services and quality of care we provide are the services and quality of care that patients want. Secondly as a **democratic** approach to ensure that health care is provided fairly, equitably and accountably. Our aim should be to increase user participation to the level where people in the local community are partners in the provision of health care rather than passive recipients.

SHARING DECISION-MAKING

Historically, the patient perspective can take one of three forms. The oldest conceptual model involves passivity on the part of the patient, and activity through the effect of one person, usually the doctor, on another, usually the patient. In this model the doctor does something to the patient: the doctor is active, the patient is passive. This situation applies, and is entirely appropriate, in the case of emergencies when the patient may be severely injured, delirious, or in a coma.

The second model underlies much of recent and existing medical practice. Although the patient may be ill, he or she is conscious and has feelings and aspirations for the encounter. Although the patient may be suffering from pain, anxiety, or other distressing symptoms, help is sought and there is a willingness to co-operate. The doctor is placed in a position of power, and it is this that distinguishes the relationship. The doctor has knowledge about the patient's bodily processes in health and illness, and possesses technical knowledge and expertise. The patient is expected to 'obey' the doctor, usually without question or disagreement. The relationship is one of guidance from the doctor and co-operation from the patient.

A more mature model, and one that more patients today are seeking, is that of mutual participation. This model is predicated on the postulation that equality among human beings is desirable. Here there is more of a partnership. The doctor certainly has expertise – but so has the patient. Not only may the patient's own experiences of the illness or disease provide reliable and important clues that can help in management, any programme of treatment often needs to be carried out by the patient. This is particularly true of chronic disorders such as diabetes, but in terms of familiarity with the effect on them, may also apply to patients experiencing even minor illnesses.

Most doctors are familiar with patients who have rare disorders. Many such patients become experts to the point where they may well have considerably greater knowledge than, perhaps, their general practitioner. This may be added to the expertise that they have relating to how the condition affects them personally.

The nature of the consultation and the relationship between the doctor and patient as a team will therefore vary. This is likely to be dependent on what each brings to any individual consultation, not only in terms of attitude, but also of style. The effectiveness of any interaction and possibly even intervention may then be highly interdependent.

However, there is always a unique potential of any consultation, originally described in relation to general practitioners (see Figure 10.9),[6] and this probably exists for any episode of patient contact with a health professional.

Clinical decision-making should increasingly be moving from a position of 'doctor knows best' to that where information about treatment options and patient choices is shared and the decision is made by the doctor and patient together. Patients are increasingly demanding better information and greater inclusion of their values and preferences into clinical decision-making. We are at a place where two rivers meet: one of increasing availability and access to knowledge, the other of empowerment and individual choice.

Limited consultation times often prevent adequate discussion of choices, but other methods can be used to share information:

- *Leaflets and videos.* These allow patients to find out about their illness and treatment choices in their own time and home environment. Although the quality of such information is variable, efforts by national organizations and patient groups have gradually improved the accuracy and value of such materials.

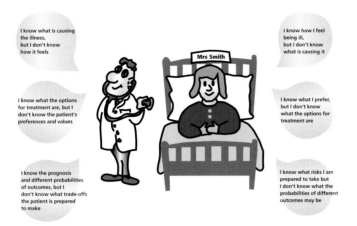

Medical care will work most effectively when both parties share their knowledge and expertise

Fig. 10.9 Medical care will work most effectively when both parties share their knowledge and expertise.

- *CD-ROMs and computer programmes.* These allow much greater scope for allowing patients to consider and explore different alternatives and may become more commonplace in health care settings.
- *Internet.* There are a huge number of health websites on the Internet, with little regulation or quality assessment. Most of us will be familiar now with patients coming to clinic armed with dubious information downloaded from the Internet. It is the nature of our information revolution that such sources will continue to expand and be used. It is unlikely that any attempt to regulate or apply quality standards will ever keep up with the expansion, or even if it did, would be valued by patients. National sites such as the NHS Direct Online aim to provide a central and reliable source of health knowledge for patients in the future.
- *Seminars and workshops.* These can provide a forum for health professionals to inform and educate patients. For patients they provide the opportunity to raise questions in a supportive environment.

TOWARDS PARTNERSHIP

We cannot expect to be taken seriously about the quality of care we provide if we do not strive to ensure that patients' views and values are given primacy. These days we talk not just about patient involvement, but about patient partnership and even patient empowerment.

Some of this discussion can appear adversarial. Some of the advocates for patient empowerment have axes to grind and prejudices about hospital doctors being relics from the days of Sir Lancelot Spratt. Professionals on the other hand harbour their own prejudices about patient partnership. In addition to a natural defensiveness about questioning of their judgement and decisions, there are inevitable pressures on time and resources that limit the feasibility of true informed decision-making.

One thing is clear however. The world is changing and health service users are becoming more informed and more demanding. Younger generations socialized as active consumers of the services they use want to know more about their choices and the risks and benefits of the medical interventions they receive. While many patients are happy to abdicate decisions and choices to the doctor, there is an ever-growing number of patients who want more say in the care and treatment that they receive.

The next step to consider is promoting partnership with patients. This can be threatening to doctors and health professionals who are used to a transactional relationship in which the patient is the child and the professional is the parent. It can be threatening to patients who prefer this type of relationship. However, the public are becoming more consumerist and aware of choices in their lives, and health, while important, is just another area of choice.

Each clinical department needs to consider how to promote patient partnership in their clinical governance arrangements. Clinical governance groups should include a user representative. User views should help dictate clinical governance priorities. Progress in quality improvement should be shared with users and disseminated widely in the local community.

As usual this is easier said than done. In reality it can be difficult to find user representatives who are confident enough to contribute in clinical groups, or who do not have personal agendas to pursue, or have the time and enthusiasm to participate. Some groups, such as care of the elderly or paediatrics, may need to involve carers more than patients. Certain groups, such as some Accident and Emergency or general surgery groups, often have brief and short-term contacts with patients and may struggle to identify candidates for longer-term involvement.

One method for promoting genuine partnership is to establish a users advisory group. This can provide a forum for debate and discussion for a diverse group of patients. Patients can be identified from a variety of sources such as community organizations and voluntary groups, rather than relying on people selected by professionals who are likely to be satisfied with the service. Efforts should be made to ensure appropriate ethnic and gender composition. The issues raised in these meetings can then be taken back to the main clinical governance group either by one of the user advisory group members or by the group facilitator.

Wider patient partnership can be pursued by the hospital through groups such as the Patient Forum and the Patient Advocacy and Liaison Service. These are patient groups established to provide greater patient representation and advocacy in health trusts.

LISTENING TO WHAT PATIENTS WANT

The traditional method of obtaining patient views has been a suggestion box on the ward or outside a clinic, often with no accompanying pen or paper, and sometimes never opened. More sophisticated methods of user involvement should be promoted and some of these are described below. Before starting any user involvement exercise it is essential that you are clear about its aims and objectives; which patients you want to involve and how you will access the hard to reach groups; what you will do with the results.

Methods include:

- *Public meetings.* These provide the opportunity for users to discuss local services and feedback their views. However, attendance may be variable and selective, and organization can be costly and time-consuming. Beware of tokenistic meetings for PR purposes.
- *Questionnaire surveys.* Can be given out on the ward or sent out by post. They provide a structured means of collecting detailed data on a large sample. Response rates may be low or biased and the quantifiable information can lack depth. Good design and administrative support will be needed.
- *Focus groups.* Usually made up of six to eight users, with a semi-structured, facilitator-led discussion on specific health topics. Participants can be randomly or purposively selected. The group environment promotes confidence in expressing opinions and a wide-ranging overview of the issues. Good facilitation is important and this can be expensive.
- *One-to-one interviews.* These can be carried out in person or by telephone. Users can be sampled randomly or purposively. Issues can be explored in great depth and can cover sensitive areas. Expertise will be required to undertake and analyse the interviews.
- *Health panels and citizens' juries.* These are groups or networks of local people that are used to provide ongoing views and feedback about local health services. They can also inform decision-making about local priorities.

All these methods require time and money. Health care organizations often just consider their costs; however, there will be costs for the participating patients and these need to be recognized and reimbursed. The costs are no excuse for delaying efforts to involve patients, just a barrier that needs to be recognized and addressed early on in the process.

WHEN THINGS GO WRONG

Despite best endeavours, things can and will go wrong. What matters then is how the individuals, teams and the organization respond. Some of these aspects are discussed in other chapters.

Learning from complaints

The NHS complaints procedure has been reformed a number of times, but concerns remain that the system remains too complicated and confusing.

Trusts must investigate and apologize to the complainant where appropriate. If the complainant is not satisfied with the outcome of the investigation, their complaint may be referred for an independent review by a panel of lay people (supported by professional advisers). Complainants also have a right to complain to the Health Service Ombudsman. The system is designed to resolve complaints without recourse to litigation.

Three times a year the office of the Health Service Ombudsman publishes details of the cases it has investigated. In these reports there is an attempt to illustrate issues that may have a general application (see Box 10.5).

Box 10.5 Complaints investigated by the Health Service Ombudsman

Inadequate care and treatment of a patient with chest pain in an A&E department

The patient attended an A&E department having developed sudden severe pain over his chest, arms and back. He was not seen by a doctor for nearly 3 hours. He was discharged but collapsed and died later that day with a ruptured dissecting aneurysm.

There had been an unacceptable delay in the doctor seeing the patient. The junior doctor who saw the patient had little experience of a relatively rare disorder. He failed to evaluate the chest pain and did not seek advice from a senior colleague as he should have done.

A man suffering from chest pains was taken by ambulance to an A&E department. He was examined and sent home. Four days later he returned to the A&E department where he was examined by an SHO. The SHO thought he had unstable angina and referred him to the medical SHO. There was a delay in the patient being seen by the medical SHO, which led to a further delay in starting anticoagulant treatment. In the early hours of the following day the patient had a fatal heart attack.

The Ombudsman found that the patient had been inappropriately discharged initially. The professional assessors advised that the delays in the patient being seen fell below an acceptable standard.

The Trust agreed that in future the decision to admit or discharge a patient with suspected cardiac pain would be made by a doctor of registrar grade or above.

The Ombudsman underlined the lesson from these two cases as being the need for adequate support and supervision of junior clinical staff, and that he had mentioned this in his previous report.

(Source: www.ombudsman.org.uk)

REFERENCES

1. Reason J. Understanding adverse events: human factors. In: Vincent C (ed) *Clinical Risk Management*. London: BMJ Publishing Group, 1995.
2 Helmreigh RL, Schaefer H-G. Team performance in the operating room. In: Bogner MS (ed) *Human Errors in Medicine*. Hillsdale, NJ: Erlbaum, 1994.
3. Report of the Inter-Departmental Committee on the Remuneration of Consultants and Specialists. London: HMSO, 1948 (Cmd 7420) (The Spens Report).
4. Belbin RM. *Management Teams: Why They Succeed or Fail*. London: Butterworth-Heinemann, 1981.
5. Irvine D. The performance of doctors. II: Maintaining good practice, protecting patients from poor performance. *BMJ* 1997; **314**: 1613–1615.
6. Stott NCH, Davis RH. The exceptional potential in each primary care consultation. *J R Coll Gen Pract* 1979; **29**: 201–205.

Working in a managed health service

In this chapter we look at:

- Developments in management
- Developments in management in the NHS
- Current management arrangements
- Management arrangements for ensuring quality
- Negligence by doctors
- Health service guidance
- The General Medical Council
- Employment arrangements
- Managing poor performance
- Management and leadership
- Effective managers
- Managing yourself
- Working with managers
- Managing change
- Efficiency and effectiveness
- Systems as the key to quality
- The learning organization.

DEVELOPMENTS IN MANAGEMENT

Up to and even beyond the 1950s management was viewed as a science. Financial numbers and hierarchical structures were seen as the way to run an organization. Organizations tended to be seen as machines that should run as efficiently as possible. In the 1960s the pendulum swung towards the organization being viewed less as a machine and more as a social system. Success was sought through helping employees realize their full potential: managing people instead of managing numbers.

In the 1970s economic recession coupled with oil crises led to the break-up of the massive companies and conglomerates that had been created. This was the time of a shift towards smaller business units. Instead of large monolithic organizations, these smaller units were thought to be more responsive to changes in the environment, such as the increasing economic challenge from Japan. In the 1980s techniques were borrowed from the Japanese. These included a range of approaches to quality, for example, total quality management (TQM) and continuous quality improvement (CQI).

More recently, in the 1990s, management thinking has been heavily influenced by perspectives that see the world as inherently unstable, with unexpected shifts and changes. These can create huge opportunities or major threats. There has been a move from national and international to global competition. Firms have struggled to remain responsive to local and national markets and circumstances, whilst at the same time looking to gain the benefits of operating globally, including economies of scale. Strategic flexibility has been the watchword, with much greater fluidity in the boundaries between organizations and the environment. The shift has been from formally linked structures to relationships and virtual organizations. There is a prevailing idea of partnership: between organizations; with the government and the public; and with their employees. However, any organization continuously changing itself as a whole would hardly ever be able to function. This has led to the notion of learning companies. A learning company is an organization that facilitates the learning of all its members and consciously transforms itself and its context; in other words it becomes efficiently adaptive in the right place at the right time and in the right way to take advantage of environmental change.

Now, knowledge is becoming the most creative force, spawning new products, services, technologies and industries, forms of communication, types of food and treatments for illness. Previously the critical assets were raw materials, land, labour and machinery. Now the raw materials are know-how, creativity, ingenuity and imagination. The new generations are the beneficiaries of unprecedented flows of knowledge from science and education. What a change! In the 1890s, critics warned that bicycle-riding would lead to an epidemic of bicycle face, a permanent disfigurement caused by pedalling into the wind at high speed.

DEVELOPMENTS IN MANAGEMENT IN THE NHS

The NHS has not been immune to these changes. However, the introduction of management theories and practice has come somewhat late in the day. By the early 1980s there were major problems with the NHS. Demand had increased to the point where the largest share of resources was being used to support the acute hospitals. Containing costs became an increasing problem. Growth and developments were occurring without proper planning.

An inquiry into the NHS was published in 1983.[1] The Griffiths Report looked at the management of the NHS and found a lack of clarity about these arrangements. In particular, accountability arrangements at a local level were unclear.

The Griffiths Report did away with management by consensus and led to the introduction of general management into the health service; it was thus an important landmark. Senior managers were appointed to lead each hospital and health authority. These managers were accountable for the performance of their organization. Doctors were gradually drawn into this process; some became medical directors and others were appointed as clinical directors. However, this accountability was largely linked with financial or workload performance, and not with the quality of the service.

In the 1990s the then Conservative Government introduced the internal market, separating the roles of purchasing and providing care. It was judged that the potential for collusion between the health authority and the hospitals it was responsible for meant that there was little incentive to improve the quality of care. In the internal market, the purchasers of care (health authorities and general practice fundholders) were separated from the providers of care, the hospitals and community services. It was intended that financial incentives and the availability of choice (as to where services were obtained) would ensure that services were purchased locally to meet the health needs of the population, and drive up their quality and the efficiency with which they were provided. Contracts between purchasers and providers made explicit how much of what was being bought, and at what quality.

In 1997 a new Labour Government abandoned the internal market. Policy documents and a white paper that led to legislation were designed to put quality at the heart of the NHS. For the first time a statutory duty of quality was introduced. The Government embarked on a 10-year plan to modernize the NHS to ensure fair access to prompt high quality care wherever a patient is treated in the NHS.[2] The NHS Plan is designed to provide a health service for the 21st century, designed around the patient. Considerable investment is included, but linked to the planned reforms. Links were made between health and social care.

The UK is one of the few places in the world where the NHS always figures prominently on the political agenda and heavily in any general election. The Department of Health is one of the biggest government ministries, with a large budget (about £40 billion in 1998/1999 and significant year on year rises after that reaching an increase in real terms of one third in 5 years), and the Secretary of State for Health is one of the most senior and sought-after Cabinet positions. The Department of Health, like any other government department, is staffed by civil servants whose job is to support their ministers and to translate government policy into health service policy, regulations and guidance.

In the 1990s, to separate the running of the NHS more clearly from policy-making, the headquarters of the NHS Executive were moved out of London and based in Leeds. There was an NHS Chief Executive and a Board.

With the abolition of Regional Health Authorities in 1996, eight regional offices of the NHS Executive were established in England, each with a Director who sits on the NHS Board. The principal role of these regional offices was on the one hand to support the roll out and implementation of NHS policy through helping and supporting NHS organizations and health professionals, and on the other to manage the performance of the NHS locally.

There were approximately 100 health authorities in England (in Scotland and Northern Ireland there are Health Boards which combine the role of health authorities and social service departments, as well as overseeing primary care). The job of these health authorities was to assess the health and health care needs of their resident population, and then to purchase or commission the provision of services to meet these needs. The mechanism for achieving this was through contracts with a range of providers, principally hospital and primary care trusts. A local Health Improvement Plan was used as the instrument for setting out what the health authority wished to achieve in the short and longer term, and these plans were produced after consultation with all interested parties, including the public.

CURRENT MANAGEMENT ARRANGEMENTS

The current structure of the NHS is being streamlined, with the abolition of the eight regional offices and the existing health authorities. These will be replaced by about 30 Strategic Health Authorities whose main role will be to take on the performance management role previously carried out by the regional offices. NHS structures will be more closely aligned with local authority arrangements. The intention is to push decision-making and associated funding right to the front line where services, it is believed, should be planned as well as delivered. The locus for this planning is being shifted to Primary Care Trusts. Primary Care Trusts are intended to put professionals in the driving seat, but also enable public involvement. They also have a duty of probity and public accountability to their health authorities.

The separation of the policy-making role of the Department of Health and the executive arm, the NHS Executive, running the NHS has always been fraught with tension. After a period of attempting greater separation in the 1990s, the two have now been brought closer together by the appointment of an NHS Chief Executive who is also the Permanent Secretary for the Department of Health (its most senior civil servant).

MANAGEMENT ARRANGEMENTS FOR ENSURING QUALITY

What mechanisms are there in place to ensure that doctors conform to the highest quality standards? Earlier chapters have set out arrangements for promoting and ensuring quality in health care, through organizations like NICE and CHAI.

Doctors, like other citizens, have a duty to comply with the law, and the sanctions for not doing so can, of course, be considerable. A number of Statutory Instruments govern the health service and the conduct of individuals working within the NHS and to all intents and purposes have the force of law.

Negligence by doctors

If a doctor has behaved negligently towards a patient, then it may be possible for the patient (or a representative) to sue the doctor for damages in a civil court. A number of conditions must be satisfied for a successful claim. The doctor must have a legal duty of care owed to that patient. The doctor's behaviour must have fallen short of the standard required by law, and it must have been reasonably foreseeable that the negligent behaviour in question could damage the patient. In a famous case (Bolam v Friern Barnet Hospital Management Committee in 1957[3,4] – see Box 11.1) it was established that if a doctor treats a patient in a way that is considered acceptable at the time by one responsible body of medical opinion, the doctor cannot be held to be negligent even if there is another responsible body of medical opinion which considers the treatment in question to be wrong. This test still stands, although the rising cost of medical litigation, and the consequent opportunity cost, is raising questions and a debate about alternative ways of helping patients who have been harmed by NHS medical care.

Health service guidance

Health service circulars, guidance or professional letters are issued by the Department of Health or the NHS Executive and also define policy, usually in more focused areas of professional work or practice. Health service circulars and guidance do not have the statutory force of law but compliance with these is expected for those working in the NHS. It would be difficult for a doctor acting with blatant disregard to such guidance to defend a different position or approach. Their weight, though, is different from guidelines and protocols, particularly those produced by eminent groups or organizations, such as the Medical Royal Colleges or specialist associations. Such documents will have the weight of a substantial and authoritative body of medical

---

Box 11.1   The standard of skill required of doctors

Mr Bolam was a patient who suffered from depressive illness. His general practitioner referred him to a consultant psychiatrist, who recommended electro-convulsive therapy. There was a school of thought which believed that muscle relaxant drugs should be used during the convulsion, with the intention of preventing the occurrence of fractures. However, the psychiatrist to whom Mr Bolam was referred belonged to a different school of thought which believed that there were side effects to the use of such drugs and that they outweighed the possible benefits. Mr Bolam duly underwent the treatment without the relaxants, but he unfortunately found that both his hips had been fractured in the process. He therefore sued the psychiatrist, together with the anaesthetist, for negligence in terms of failure to use the muscle relaxants.

The action failed.

'When you get a situation which involves the use of some special skill or competence, then the test as to whether there has been negligence is not the test of the man on the top of the Clapham Omnibus because he has not got this special skill. The test is the standard of the ordinary skilled man exercising and professing to have that special skill.'

'A doctor is not guilty of negligence if he has acted in accordance with the practice accepted as proper by a responsible body of medical men skilled in that particular art ... Putting it the other way round, a doctor is not negligent if he is acting in accordance with such a practice merely because there is a body of opinion that takes a contrary view.'

Trial judge: McNair J

(Bolam v Friern Hospital Management Committee (1957). In: Scott W. *The General Practitioner & The Law of Negligence*. London: Cavendish, 1994.)

opinion, and are designed to be helpful to practitioners in practising evidence-based health care. However, they may be considered as only one 'body of opinion' among others (see above).

For some areas of health care (currently including cancer, coronary heart disease, mental health, the care of older people, and the care of children) National Service Frameworks have been issued. These set standards and targets, as well as describing models of best practice, i.e. benchmarking (see Chapter 1).

The General Medical Council

Doctors also have additional codes of conduct to observe.

The essential character of a profession is that its members have specialized knowledge and skills which the public will wish to use. The public therefore have an interest in being able to recognize a qualified practitioner and will wish to be provided with a register of qualified individuals. Any such register must list only those with a certain standard of competence. The body responsible for maintaining the register will therefore have two duties to discharge. First, it will have to assure itself that those admitted to the register are competent. Second, it will have to remove those practitioners who are unfit to practise. The maintenance of a register of the competent is fundamental to the regulation of a profession.

This theory was turned into practice for the medical profession in the UK by the Medical Act of 1958, by which the General Medical Council (GMC) was established. The duty of the GMC is to protect the public as well as supporting doctors.

More recently the statute governing the registration of medical practitioners has been the Medical Act 1983. However, in the wake of a number of serious cases of malpractice, public and governmental pressures are leading to reforms with further changes to the statutes. Modernization of the GMC, along with the modernization of the NHS, is well underway.

The GMC has the power to suspend, or alter the conditions of, registration. They are routinely notified of criminal convictions of doctors, and registration may be suspended if a doctor is found guilty of serious professional misconduct. In future revalidation will be necessary every 5 years to ensure continued registration and the right to practise.

The GMC has set out clear standards covering the general context of medical practice.[5] Specialist areas of practice are set out in a wide range of policy documents published by the Medical Royal Colleges and specialist associations. Doctors are expected to conform with these explicit and clear standards for professional practice.

Employment arrangements

Most hospital doctors in the NHS are also employees, and are thus governed by their contracts of employment. There is a range of duties and expectations for both employees and employers, and doctors will similarly be expected to comply with these. With the statutory duty for clinical governance comes an

> **Box 11.2   The seven attributes of 'Good Medical Practice'**
>
> - Good clinical care
> - Maintaining good medical practice
> - Teaching and training
> - Maintaining trust
> - Working with colleagues
> - Probity
> - Health
>
> (Source: General Medical Council, 2001)

increasing level of explicit expectations for doctors to comply with risk management systems and processes, including conforming with accepted guidelines. This is given additional focus with the development of appraisal and performance review, linked to more detailed job plans and personal development plans (PDPs).

Managing poor performance

Good Medical Practice, published by the GMC,[5] defines the attributes and performance expected professionally of a doctor (see Box 11.2). If there are concerns about a doctor's fitness to practise then referral to the GMC is obligatory. The GMC has a set of performance procedures to carry out a rigorous assessment and take action, including erasure from the register, as necessary.

If there are concerns about a doctor's performance but these fall short of concerns about fitness to practise, then the doctor can be referred to the National Clinical Assessment Authority (NCAA). Whilst the procedures of this organization are still being developed, it is likely that the NCAA will commission a detailed assessment, the outcome of which may be:

- a recommendation that the doctor should be allowed to continue practice unhindered
- suggestions for limitations of the context in which the doctor may practice, e.g. certain support staff or facilities might be necessary; or
- a recommendation for further specific training.

Other aspects of performance, such as attitude or manner with colleagues or patients, may be dealt with as aspects of personal conduct, under employer disciplinary processes.

MANAGEMENT AND LEADERSHIP

Management responsibilities for doctors inevitably involve increasing tension between individual care for patients and the need for a service, as well as delivery of government priorities and objectives. It is important here to separate out the difference between professional, leadership, and management.

Working in a managed health service

187

Box 11.3   Leadership qualities

- Courage
- Desire, i.e. the strong wish to lead
- Emotional stamina – the ability to persist in the face of disappointment
- Physical stamina
- Empathy – including sensitivity to other people's values and other cultures, beliefs and traditions
- Decisiveness
- Anticipation
- Timing
- Competitiveness
- Self-confidence
- Accountability – in particular, never heaping praise on oneself for one's own achievements or laying blame on others for what one fails to achieve
- Responsibility
- Credibility
- Tenacity
- Dependability
- Stewardship – leaders are custodians of the interests and well-being of those they serve as leaders
- Loyalty

(Adapted from: Roberts W. In the Roman Court: leadership qualities. In: Syrett M, Hogg C (eds) *Frontiers of Leadership.* Oxford: Blackwell, 1992.)

There continues to be much debate about the differences between leadership and management. It is perhaps best to think of leadership as being about direction, while management is about speed, coordination (for going in the right, leader-determined, direction) and logistics. One author of an essay on leadership identified 17 qualities for a leader (see Box 11.3). What is striking is that he put these qualities into the mouth of Attila the Hun!

More recently ideas around leadership have moved towards the notion of transformational leaders. Such leaders are seen as engaging the commitment of employees in the context of shared values and a shared vision. This is particularly relevant in the context of managing change, such as has affected the health service in recent years. Transformational leaders are judged to share a number of common characteristics (see Box 11.4).

Effective managers

Effective managers, indeed effective people, have a number of characteristics which have been defined. One popular approach describes the seven habits of highly effective people (see Box 11.5).

Managing yourself

Anyone who wishes to improve the way they manage others must first learn to manage themselves. There is a large literature on various aspects of self-management.

Box 11.4   Characteristics of transformational leaders

Transformational leaders:

- Clearly see themselves as *change agents*. They set out to make a difference and to transform the organization for which they are responsible.
- Are *courageous*. They can deal with resistance, take a stand, take risks, confront reality.
- *Believe in people*. They have well-developed beliefs about motivation, trust and empowerment.
- Are driven by a strong set of *values*.
- Are lifelong *learners*. They view mistakes – their own as well as other people's – as learning opportunities.
- Can cope with *complexity, uncertainty* and *ambiguity*.
- Are *visionaries*.

(Adapted from: Tichy NM, Devanna MA. *The Transformational Leader.* New York: Wiley, 1986.)

Box 11.5   The seven habits of highly effective people

- Take responsibility for your own life
- Begin with the end in mind, including doing the right thing, and doing things right
- Put first things first (the urgent versus the important)
- Seek solutions so that everyone can win ('win–win')
- Seek first to understand, then to be understood (communication)
- Creative cooperation leading to synergy (two sides come together to produce a solution better than either side proposed)
- Self-renewal (self-maintenance and self-care: 'sharpening the saw')

(Adapted from: Covey SR. *The Seven Habits of Highly Effective People.* London: Simon & Schuster, 1999.)

One model that is helpful in managing aspects of work, for instance, papers and reports, considers the dimensions of urgency and importance (see Box 11.6).

Box 11.6   Urgency and importance

1	2
Urgent and Important	Not urgent and Important
3	**4**
Urgent and Not important	Not urgent and Not important

WORKING WITH MANAGERS

It is easy to be cynical about meetings. Meetings seem to attract high levels of satire and derision; although many people still try to impress with packed diaries full of meetings they 'have to' attend. However, meetings seem to play an increasingly critical role. Despite this, many meetings are poorly prepared, badly managed, and ineffectively concluded.

Meetings tend to reflect the organizational environment in which they are held. Meetings may have many roles, including:

- Exercising control
- Communication, both up and down
- Making decisions
- Avoiding making decisions or taking responsibility
- Achieving the organizational goals
- Sharing perspectives
- A focus on particular tasks or processes
- Achieving and managing unanimity.

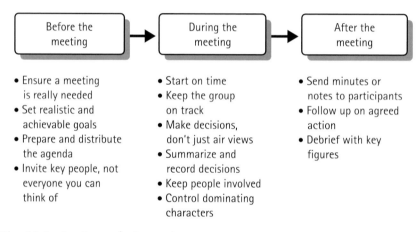

Fig. 11.1   Running productive meetings.

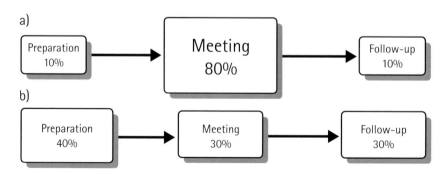

Fig. 11.2   Making meetings more productive. (a) Meetings with most of the effort concentrated on the meeting itself. (b) For more productive or key meetings, much more work needs to be put into preparation and follow-up action.

There are three main phases involved in running a productive meeting (see Figure 11.1). Meetings tend to be seen as single events, with a little preparation (perhaps 10% of the effort), most of the effort (say 80%) concentrating on the meeting itself, and perhaps 10% of effort put into follow-up action. Meeting productivity can, however, improve when much more work is done before and after the meeting (Figure 11.2).

MANAGING CHANGE

Change seems to be perpetually inflicted on the NHS; too much change can be distracting. Requirements for successful change include:

- Top management commitment
- Constant and consistent communication
- Employee involvement at all levels
- A shared vision of the future
- Understanding of the need for change
- Management of networks.

Where change is directed towards process improvement, then a self-reinforcing cycle may be started. The improvements made may create opportunities for staff. Whether in a changing environment or not, most of our interactions with people (patients and colleagues) are negotiations. This ought to mean that we all have highly developed negotiation skills. The principles of good negotiation, 'win–win' in the jargon, are not particularly difficult, and have been well set out (see Box 11.7).[6] Like all skills, the skills of negotiation can take time to acquire, practise and assimilate into regular or routine use, including with patients.

EFFICIENCY AND EFFECTIVENESS

It is useful to distinguish between some of the central terms in use in relation to quality in the NHS.[7]

Box 11.7   Getting to yes: negotiating without giving in

Any method of negotiation must:

- Produce a wise agreement if agreement is possible
- Be efficient
- Improve, or at least not damage, the relationship between the parties

Successful negotiation:

- Separates the people from the problem
- Focuses on interests, not positions
- Involves inventing options for mutual gain
- Reaches a solution on the basis of objective criteria

(Adapted from: Fisher R, Ury W. *Getting to Yes: Negotiating Agreement Without Giving In*. London: Arrow Books, 1987.)

Efficacy means the production of health benefits as demonstrated within a clinical trial. Here service delivery is rigorously controlled by the application of strict patient entry criteria, and careful targeting and monitoring of the service delivered.

Effectiveness means the production of health benefits for patients when the intervention is in general use.

Cost represents the value of what is forgone to society when an intervention or a service is provided. This is known as the opportunity cost. It should be noted that the cost to society is not equal to the charge made for an intervention. The price of a service rarely bears much relationship to its social opportunity. For example, the cost of the time of a patient is rarely counted. Nevertheless, an important point for doctors and other health professionals is that resources used in one way are not available for use in another way or for another patient. Such resources not only include money (as exemplified by the cost of a prescription or a laboratory test or X-ray), but also time. Within an organization it is also commonly held that people are its biggest resource. Cost-effectiveness is measured in terms of the production of health benefits for patients at least cost.

Much of the focus of recent administrations has been on the efficiency and effectiveness of the NHS, with considerable political and public attention devoted to these matters. Many of the changes introduced in the last decade have been attempts to obtain better value for money as well as increased efficiency. Efficiency comes from people in the organization's operational parts having appropriate authority and responsibility delegated to them so that they have the commitment and discretion to do their jobs well. They can take pride in being efficient, and are then less likely to resent being stretched by challenging targets. Effectiveness comes from senior managers and directors putting time aside to do a decent job of monitoring the external environment, debating and discussing issues, and reframing them. In this way the organization can always be attuned to social, technological and political change, giving it more freedom to shape its future.

SYSTEMS AS THE KEY TO QUALITY

We have looked at some of the issues relating to the individual performance of the doctor (or for that matter other health professionals). It is important to recognize that the great majority of adverse events in the NHS are not indicative of or attributable to deep-seated problems of poor performance on the part of individual clinicians.[8] Currently there is a range of systems for gaining information about and learning from adverse events (see Box 11.8), but these have a number of weaknesses.[8] Steps are therefore in hand to re-think the way that the NHS approaches the challenge of learning from adverse health care events. This work includes looking at unified mechanisms for reporting and analysis when things go wrong; a more open culture, in which errors or service failures can be reported and discussed; mechanisms for ensuring that, where lessons are identified, the necessary changes are put into practice; and the need to develop a much wider appreciation of the value of the systems

---

Box 11.8   Current NHS systems providing information on adverse events

- Incident reporting systems (e.g. local risk reporting systems in NHS Trusts; untoward incident schemes run in NHS regions; reporting of adverse reactions to drugs or medical devices)
- Data derived as a by-product of systems designed to investigate or respond to instances of poor quality (e.g. litigation for alleged medical negligence; the NHS complaints procedure; cases referred to the Health Services Commissioner)
- Databases of ongoing studies on a national basis which aim to identify poor outcomes and avoidable factors in certain specific fields of health care (e.g. the national confidential enquiries in perioperative deaths, maternal mortality, stillbirth and infant deaths, homicides and suicides by mentally ill people)
- Periodic external studies and reviews (e.g. those conducted and published by the Audit Commission)
- Spontaneous reporting outside normal channels by individual members of staff ('whistleblowing')
- Health service and public health statistics

---

approach in preventing, analysing and learning from errors. It is clear that the quality that is sought through clinical governance will depend on and only be achieved through detailed attention to the health service systems. The details of many of these have been discussed in earlier chapters.

THE LEARNING ORGANIZATION

A learning organization has been described as one that facilitates the learning of all its members and consciously transforms itself and its context, thus becoming an efficient adaptive unit.[9] The idea of learning organizations is not entirely new but has evolved out of progress beyond the idea of survival of the fittest. It is the notion that an organization can be created that is capable of changing, developing and transforming itself in response to the needs and aspirations of the staff within it and, for the NHS, the patients without it.

Learning organizations have been viewed as having certain characteristics (see Box 11.9). Such organizations are about seeing, thinking and doing things differently. But they are also about being clear where responsibilities, rights

---

Box 11.9   Characteristics of a learning organization

Characteristics of the learning organization include:

- having an explicit approach to quality assurance, linked to the goals of the organization
- the development of leadership skills among staff
- valuing education and training
- an open and participative culture
- teamwork as a routine in practice
- a well-developed infrastructure which supports individual performance

---

and duties rest within an organization. The full participation of people in such an organization must lead to joint ownership and joint responsibilities.

CONCLUSION

To be responsive to change, a child, adult, organization, even society, must be adept at learning. It has been argued that organizations can only be effective if the people that run them are capable of two key skills: learning continuously and giving direction (leadership).

We have tried to show that quality is every doctor's business, consistent with the highest standards of professional practice both as currently defined, for example by the General Medical Council, and consistent with the ideals in the original Hippocratic Oath (see Box 11.10). Similarly, we have looked at the duty for quality owed by NHS organizations and their systems. This requires commitment to clinical governance from individual doctors and all health service organizations.

'Increasing our skill and our ability to treat patients is a lifelong fascinating journey. Understanding the interrelationship between the patient and his disease and the effects of the social, economic and physical environment is a never-ending quest and gratification. No physician can ask more of his destiny. Nor should he be satisfied with less.'[10]

Working in a managed health service

Box 11.10   The Oath by Hippocrates

I swear by Apollo the physician, and Aesculapius, and Health, and All-heal, and all the gods and goddesses, that, according to my ability and judgement, I will keep this Oath and this stipulation to reckon him who taught me this Art equally dear to me as my parents, to share my substance with him, and relieve his necessities if required; to look upon his offspring in the same footing as my own brothers, and to teach them this art, if they shall wish to learn it, without fee or stipulation; and that by precept, lecture, and every other mode of instruction, I will impart a knowledge of the Art to my own sons, and those of my teachers, and to disciples bound by a stipulation and oath according to the law of medicine, but to none others. I will follow that system of regimen which, according to my ability and judgement, I consider for the benefit of my patients, and abstain from whatever is deleterious and mischievous. I will give no deadly medicine to any one if asked, nor suggest any such counsel; and in like manner I will not give to a woman a pessary to produce abortion. With purity and with holiness I will pass my life and practice my Art. I will not cut persons laboring under the stone, but will leave this to be done by men who are practitioners of this work. Into whatever houses I enter, I will go into them for the benefit of the sick, and will abstain from every voluntary act of mischief and corruption; and, further from the seduction of females or males, of freemen and slaves. Whatever, in connection with my professional practice or not, in connection with it, I see or hear, in the life of men, which ought not to be spoken of abroad, I will not divulge, as reckoning that all such should be kept secret. While I continue to keep this Oath unviolated, may it be granted to me to enjoy life and the practice of the art, respected by all men, in all times! But should I trespass and violate this Oath, may the reverse be my lot!

(Written 400 BCE. Translated by Francis Adams. From: *http://classics.mit.edu/Hippocrates/hippoath.html*)

1. Griffiths R. *NHS Management Enquiry*. London: Department of Health and Social Security, 1983.
2. Department of Health. *The NHS Plan: A Plan for Investment; A Plan For Reform*. London: Department of Health, 2000.
3. Scott W. *The General Practitioner & The Law of Negligence*. London: Cavendish, 1994.
4. Irwin S, Fazan C, Allfrey R. *Medical Negligence Litigation: A Practitioner's Guide*. London: Legal Action Group, 1995.
5. GMC. *Good Medical Practice*. London: General Medical Council, 2001.
6. Fisher R, Ury W. *Getting to Yes: Negotiating Agreement without Giving In*. London: Arrow Books, 1987.
7. Bloor K, Maynard A. *Clinical Governance: Clinician, Heal Thyself?* London: Institute of Health Services Management, 1998.
8. Department of Health. *An Organisation with a Memory*: Report of an expert group on learning from adverse events in the NHS chaired by the Chief Medical Officer. London: The Stationery Office, 2000.
9. Pedler M, Burgoyne J, Boydell T. *The Learning Company: A Strategy for Sustainable Development*. London: McGraw-Hill, 1997.
10. Fox T. Purposes of medicine. *Lancet* 1965; **ii**: 801–805.

Working in a managed health service

APPENDIX

REVIEW ISSUES

Patient experience

Clinical effectiveness and outcomes
1. Mortality rates following admission and treatment
2. Evidence of morbidity following admission and treatment
3. Evidence of effective/ineffective practice
4. Evidence of competence/incompetence

Access to services
5. Physical access; bus services; car parks; location
6. Responsiveness; waiting times and lists
7. Disablement, ethnicity, poverty
8. Range of services in relation to need

Organization of care
9. Experience of admission of care episode
10. Experience of diagnosis of care episode
11. Experience of treatment stage of care episode
12. Experience of discharge of care episode

Humanity of care
13. Privacy and confidentiality
14. Patient involvement in their own care, e.g. information and communication
15. Promoting well being, e.g. advice and support for independent living
16. Delivery of care; respect and dignity; staff attitudes; mixed sex wards/ toilets

The environment
17. Physical state of facilities
18. Catering

Strategic capacity

1. Leadership
2. Accountabilities and structures
3. Direction and planning
4. Health economy partnerships
5. Patient and public partnerships
6. Performance review

Note: The dimensions of strategic capacity listed above are temporary and will be replaced when assessment of strategic capacity begins in reviews (planned for April 2002). At that time, a substructure of issues beneath each dimension will be introduced.

Components

Patient/service user and public involvement

Accountabilities and structures

1. Committee responsibilities for patient/service user/carer and public involvement.
2. Staff responsibilities for patient/service user/carer and public involvement work.
3. Reporting and monitoring – to/by management teams, committees and the board, e.g. of trends in patient/service user-initiated areas of concern and complaints.

Strategies and plans

4. Strategy and implementation plans for patient/service user and public involvement work.
5. Connection of the strategy with wider clinical governance and quality improvement programmes.
6. Involvement of patient/service users/carers, or their representative organizations, in policy and planning of services, e.g. through public participation groups; citizen juries; stakeholder conferences; lay/citizen and patient/service user/carer representation on Board and clinical governance committees.
7. Involvement of partners in strategy development and implementation plans.
8. Resources (staff and budget) to support the implementation of the strategy for patient/service user and public involvement.

Application of policies, strategies and plans

9. Information to the wider public about what the organization is doing, e.g. communications work, reporting on involvement work; and how well it is doing, e.g. performance information.
10. 'Customer' care practice to ensure patient/service users' privacy, dignity and confidentiality about themselves and their treatment, e.g. codes of conduct; attitudes and behaviours of staff.

11. Availability and quality of written or other information for patient/service users about treatments, services and facilities.
12. Involvement of patient/service users or carers in treatment choices, including processes for patient/service users to consent to treatment.
13. Arrangements to meet patients/service users' particular needs, e.g. cultural, dietary.
14. Access by patient/service users to information about their care, e.g. shared care plans; patient-held records; copies of correspondence between health professionals.
15. Arrangements for patient/service user/carers to voice concerns, issues and compliments about services, e.g. comment cards; suggestion boxes.
16. Systems for individual patient/service user and carers to seek redress, e.g. complaints system; PALS; Independent Complaints Advisory Service.

Quality improvements and learning
17. Involvement of patient/service users, carers and the public in monitoring the quality of care, e.g. research into patient/service user/carers' views; monitoring and evaluation of services from patient/service user/carers' perspectives.
18. Analysis of all feedback (including complaints) from individual patient/service users on their experience of the organization.
19. Improvements to the quality of service outcomes (performance) and to the quality of decision making (governance) as a result of patient/service user involvement work.
20. Dissemination of lessons learnt from consultation and patient/service user involvement activities.

Resources and training for staff
21. Training for staff in patient/service user (customer) care; communication skills; obtaining patient/service users' consent to treatment; confidentiality issues; complaints handling.
22. Support for individual patient/service users, e.g. patients' advocates; support for carers; interpreters; translation services; signers; link workers, 'expert patient' support schemes.

Clinical audit

Accountabilities and structures
1. Committee structure for clinical audit.
2. Staff responsibilities for clinical audit.
3. Reporting and monitoring – to/by management teams, committees and the board.

Strategies and plans
4. Strategy for clinical audit – including priority given to participation in national, regional and local audits – and programmes.

5. Integration of clinical audit with quality improvement programmes, e.g. to audit compliance with evidence-based practice protocols, guidelines and care pathways, etc.
6. Involvement of patient/service users and carers in clinical audit strategy and programme development.
7. Involvement of partners in cross-organizational clinical audit.
8. Support and resources for clinical audit including:
   - central clinical audit unit to support audit design, data collection and analysis
   - budgets for clinical audits

Application of policies, strategies and plans
9. Clinical audits carried out including:
   - connections with other clinical governance activities
   - staff awareness and involvement
10. Participation in national confidential enquiries.

Quality improvements and learning
11. Processes to consider the results of clinical audits.
12. Compliance with evidence-based practice shown by audits.
13. Quality improvements as a result of clinical audits.
14. Dissemination of lessons learnt from clinical audit.

Resources and training for staff
15. Training and development for staff in audit skills.

Risk management

Accountabilities and structures
1. Committee structure for clinical risk management.
2. Staff responsibilities for risk management.
3. Reporting and monitoring – to/by management teams, committees and the board.

Strategies and plans
4. Strategy and implementation plans for risk management.
5. Integration of all risk management activities (clinical, non-clinical, health and safety).
6. Integration of risk management with audit and quality improvement programmes.
7. Consideration of risk in decision-making processes.
8. Involvement of patients, service users and carers in risk management.
9. Involvement of partners in developing risk management strategies where risk is to patients/service users who are cared for by more than one organization, e.g. other health organizations, social services, police.
10. Resources for risk management including:
    - Budgets for risk management activities

- Specialist teams and support, e.g. for infection control and pressure sore control and tissue viability

Application of policies, strategies and plans
11. Risk assessment, including:
    - the collation of information from all sources about risks and monitoring of incidents and trends
    - inclusion of information from patient/service users (e.g. from complaints)
    - involvement of partners, e.g. at discharge meetings for users at risk
12. Incident and near-miss reporting and investigation.
13. Risk management, including use of trigger events, protocols.
14. Prevention and control of specific risks, e.g. misuse of drugs; use of medical devices; lone workers; infections; pressure sores; violence/self harm.

Quality improvements and learning
15. Analysis of individual risks and events and trends.
16. Quality improvements as a result of risk management activities.
17 Dissemination of lessons learnt from risk management activities.

Resources and training for staff
18. Training and education for staff in risk prevention and management.

Education, training and continuing personal and professional development

Accountabilities and structures
1. Committee structure for education, training and CPD issues.
2. Staff responsibilities education, training and CPD.
3. Reporting and monitoring – to/by management teams, committees and the board.

Strategies and plans
4. Strategy and plans for education, training and CPD.
5. Links between training and CPD programmes and wider quality improvement programmes, and with individuals' personal development plans.
6. Partnerships with educational establishments; joint training programmes with partners, e.g. other health organizations, social services, police.
7. Budget for professional development, education and training (excluding SIFT and MADEL).

Application of policies, strategies and plans
8. Personal development planning
9. Mandatory training, including CPR; manual handling
10. Work-based training schemes

11. CPD programmes
12. Schemes for obtaining relevant professional, or further, qualifications

Quality improvements and learning
13. Improvements to services and facilities following external assessments (e.g. by Royal Colleges) and internal evaluations of training and education programmes.
14. Dissemination of knowledge of effective education, training and CPD methods.

Resources and training for staff
15. Time, financial and other support for staff undergoing formal education and for individuals' CPD activities.

Clinical effectiveness programmes

Accountabilities and structures
1. Committee responsibilities for clinical effectiveness programmes.
2. Staff responsibilities for clinical effectiveness programmes.
3. Reporting and monitoring of implementation of, and compliance with, evidence-based practice – to/by management teams, committees and the board.

Strategies and plans
4. Strategy and programmes for clinical effectiveness work, including research to identify effective clinical practice.
5. Coordination of clinical effectiveness strategy and programmes with the wider clinical governance and quality improvement programmes.
6. Involvement of partners in clinical effectiveness strategy development and programmes.
7. Involvement of patient/service users and carers in clinical effectiveness strategy development and programmes.
8. Resources (staff and budget) to support research, development and implementation of the effective clinical practice.

Application of policies, strategies and plans
9. Collection and distribution of evidence-based practice to the relevant teams and staff, including:
   - results of the organization's own research
   - published evidence of effective practice, including NSFs and guidance issued by NICE
10. Research projects to identify effective clinical practice.
11. Implementation and application of effective clinical practice, e.g. integrated care pathways; evidence-based guidelines for disease management.
12. Monitoring the effectiveness and application of evidence-based practice, e.g. cycle of data collection; use of performance indicators; clinical audit; team discussion; guideline amendment.

Quality improvements and learning

13. Improvements to the patient/service user experience as a result of the implementation of evidence-based practice.
14. Dissemination of learning from the implementation of evidence-based practice.

Resources and training for staff

15. Accessibility of research results and evidence of effective practice, e.g. libraries; internet; journals; intranet (or other local electronic library).
16. Training for staff, e.g. in critical appraisal skills; literature, database and internet search skills.

Staffing and staff management

Accountabilities and structures

1. Committee structure for staffing issues.
2. Staff responsibilities for staffing.
3. Reporting and monitoring – to/by management teams, committees and the board.

Strategies and plans

4. Strategy and workforce planning for staffing including:
   - delivery of national priorities including targets in Working Together and Improving Working Lives
   - links to service plans
   - current and future number requirements; skill requirements
5. Joint approaches to staffing with partner organizations, including compatible systems, e.g. with social services.

Application of policies, strategies and plans

6. HR employment processes, e.g.
   - equality of opportunity
   - good race relations
   - checking qualifications and registration
   - disciplinary and grievance procedures
7. Workplace induction
8. Individuals' performance appraisal
9. Clinical supervision and mentoring schemes
10. Systems for dealing with cases of poor performance (including procedures for whistle blowing).
11. Deployment of appropriate staffing and skills, e.g.
    - minimum 'safe' numbers and mix
    - schemes of delegation and supervision
    - protocols for staff working in extended roles (e.g. nurse prescribing)
12. Compliance with working time directives.
13. Assessment and management of risk to staff, e.g. violence to staff; workplace health and safety.

Quality improvements and learning
14. Systems for staff feedback, e.g. from staff attitude surveys; staff appraisal processes; exit interviews.
15. Consideration of feedback from staff and improvements to the patient/service user experience as a result.
16. Dissemination of lessons learnt from staff feedback.

Resources and training for staff
17. Employee support services, e.g.
    - occupational health services
    - independent confidential advice services
    - support against bullying and harassment

Use of information to support clinical governance and health care delivery

Accountabilities and structures
1. Committee responsibilities for information, management and technology (IM&T)
2. Staff responsibilities for IM&T
3. Reporting and monitoring of performance targets and achievements–to/by management teams, committees and the board.

Strategies and plans
4. Strategy and plans for IM&T.
5. Priority given to IM&T in strategic plans for clinical governance and to the needs of clinical governance in strategic plans for IM&T.
6. Identification of the clinical and other information needed by the Board, executive team, management teams, and clinical teams to support clinical governance and health care delivery.
7. Involvement of patients in identifying information needs.
8. Involvement of partner organizations in IM&T (e.g. LIS strategy).
9. Resources (staff and budget) to support the implementation of the IM&T strategy.

Application of policies, strategies and plans
10. Information used:
    - to monitor performance and outcomes
    - to support performance review and improvement
    - to inform clinical governance activities
    - to support implementation of policies and guidelines, e.g. Mental Health Act
11. Information management systems (including links to enable sharing of information with staff from other organizations).
12. Health care records systems, including electronic patient/service user records (including communication of patient information with staff from other organizations).
13. Processes to ensure confidentiality of information about patient/service users, e.g Caldicott guardianship; application of Data Protection Act.

14. Process and systems for assuring data quality.

Quality improvements and learning
15. Use of information to review and improve clinical practice, e.g. clinical indicators.
16. Dissemination of methods of effective use of information.

Resources and training for staff
17. Training and support for staff in the interpretation and use of clinical information.
18. Analytic support to users of information.

Glossary

SOURCES OF CLINICAL EVIDENCE AND EFFECTIVENESS

Bandolier   *http://www.jr2.ox.ac.uk/bandolier/*
Bandolier, Pain Relief, The Churchill, Headington, Oxford OX3 7LJ, UK

Best Evidence 4 database   *http://www.bmjpg.com/template.cfm?name=bmjhome*
BMJ Publishing, BMA House, Tavistock Square, London WC1H 9JR

Clinical Evidence   *http://www.clinicalevidence.org*
BMJ Publishing, BMA House, Tavistock Square, London WC1H 9JR

Cochrane Collaboration   *http://www.cochrane.de*

Cochrane Library
http://www.nelh.nhs.uk/

Update Software, Summertown Pavilion, Middle Way, Oxford OX2 7LG
http://www.update-software.com/cochrane/cochrane-frame.html

Health Evidence Bulletins Wales
http://hebw.uwcm.ac.uk/

National Coordinating Centre for Health Technology Assessment (NCCHTA)   *http://www.hta.nhsweb.nhs.uk/*

National Electronic Library for Health (NeLH)
http://www.nhs.uk/nelh/

National Institute for Clinical Excellence (NICE)
http://www.nice.org.uk/nice-web/

Netting the evidence
http://www.shef.ac.uk/~scharr/ir/netting

NHS Centre for Reviews and Dissemination (NHS CRD)
http://www.york.ac.uk/inst/crd
DARE, NHS Economic Evaluation Database, HTA database, Effective Health Care bulletins and Effectiveness Matters. NHS Centre for Reviews and Dissemination, University of York, York YO10 5DD

Ovid Evidence-Based Medicine Reviews
http://www.ovid.com/
Ovid Technologies Ltd, 107 Hammersmith Grove, London W6 0NQ

PubMed
http://www.ncbi.nlm.nih.gov/entrez/query.fcgi

OTHER USEFUL INTERNET RESOURCES

British Journal of Clinical Governance *www.emerald-library.com*

British Medical Journal *www.bmj.com*

Commission for Health Audit and Inspection *www.chai.nhs.uk*

Department of Health *www.doh.gov.uk*
National guidance on consent, including model consent forms, can be found at: *www.doh.gov.uk/consent*

Doctors net *www.doctors.net*

General Medical Council *www.gmc-uk.org*

Conference of Postgraduate Medical Deans of the UK *www.copmed.org.uk*

National Patient Safety Association (NPSA)
http://www.npsa.org.uk/index2.htm

COLLEGES

Royal College of Anaesthetists, Professional Standards Committee, 48–49 Russell Square, London WC1B 4JY
Tel: 020 7813 1900; URL: *www.rcoa.ac.uk/menu6.html*

Royal College of General Practitioners, Clinical and Special Projects Network, 14 Princes Gate, Hyde Park, London SW7 1PU
Tel: 020 7581 3232; URL: *www.rcgp.org.uk/clinspec/index.asp*

and

Royal College of General Practitioners, Effective Clinical Practice Unit, University of Sheffield, Regent Court, 30 Regent House, Sheffield S1 4DA
Tel: 0114 222 0811

Royal College of Obstetricians & Gynaecologists, Audit Unit, 27 Sussex Place, London NW1 4RG
Tel: 020 7772 6200; URL: *www.rcog.org.uk*

Royal College of Ophthalmologists, Audit Department, 17 Cornwall Terrace, London NW1 4QW
Tel: 020 7935 0702; URL: *www.rcophth.ac.uk/*

Royal College of Paediatrics and Child Health, Research Division, 50 Hallam Street, London W1N 6DR
Tel: 020 7307 5674; URL: *www.rcpch.ac.uk*

Royal College of Pathologists, Clinical Audit and Effectiveness, 2 Carlton House Terrace, London SW1Y 5AF
Tel: 020 7451 6732; URL: *www.rcpath.org/activities/audit.html*

Royal College of Physicians, Clinical Effectiveness and Evaluation Unit, 11 St Andrew's Place, London NW1 4LE
Tel: 020 7935 1174; URL: *www.rcplondon.ac.uk/college.ceeu_home.htm*

Royal College of Psychiatrists, College Research Unit, 17 Belgrave Square, London SW1X 8PG
Tel: 020 7235 2351, Ext 234; URL: *www.rcpsych.ac.uk/cru*

Royal College of Radiologists, Clinical Audit Advisor, 38 Portland Place, London W1N 4JQ
Tel: 020 7636 4432; URL: *www.rcr.ac.uk*

Royal College of Surgeons of England, Clinical Effectiveness Unit, 35–43 Lincoln's Inn Fields, London WC2A 3PN
Tel: 020 7869 6600; URL: *www.rcseng.ac.uk/public/ceu/default.asp*

Glossary

Index

Index